# AWESOME AGAIN

Seven Simple Steps
for a Man to Regain His Vitality

FLAVIO BALLERINI, PH.D

**INCLUDES GUIDED MEDITATIONS
TO INSTALL THE
SEVEN STEPS
TO AWESOMENESS
IN YOUR SUBCONSCIOUS MIND**

ISBN: 978-1-951028-35-0

# DEDICATION

This book is dedicated to my True Teachers,
the thousands of clients and students who taught me the
meaning of giving, and to my four daughters, who are
teaching me the meaning of love. I thank each one
of you from the bottom of my heart.

# YOUR PERSONAL PORTAL

In your personal portal, you will find the guided meditations that will install the Seven Steps to become Awesome Again in your subconscious mind for permanent change for the better.

I thank you for purchasing this book and include the guided meditations in your personal portal as part of this book with no extra cost to you.

**To enter your personal portal, go to:**
**www.flaviolife.com/aa**

# TABLE OF CONTENTS

# ACKNOWLEDGMENTS

I feel so much gratitude for so many people who had something to do with this book that I know it would not be practical to mention them all here or to explain how much they contributed. Still, I would like to introduce you to a few people who are important to me.

My parents invested in my education, which is a big part of my life. I had the opportunity to thank them in person on several occasions for their generosity.

Mary, my first wife, gave me two beautiful daughters, Sophia and Isis, whom I love so dearly. Years after our divorce, when I was most broken, you stood by me, believed in me, and probably saved my life. I am eternally grateful to you!

The babies, my second two daughters, Solange and Mariana, you inspire me so much! Both of you are teaching Papi the meaning of love on a whole different scale. Thank you Bebes!

My buddies stood by me during my worst moments. When I was not sure I could "go on" they stood up and asked how they could help. Thank you, Misael Crespo, Reynaldo Gomez, Giuliano Boreggio, Miguel Guibert, Cristobal Herrera, Daniel Lugo, and Yazniel Meana. For sure, this book would not exist without all of you.

Marcia Dunn is such a kind soul. I have known Marcia for many years, and each time I have seen her, she has left me better and more inspired than before. Marcia came to a class once; the next day, she told me: you really should write that book. Marcia, coming from you, it meant a lot to me; here it is, and thank you for believing!

My friends Luz Elena Mora, Janet Hoyos, and Carolina Ospina are so kind to me that I actually think of them as angels. Thank you for the untold number of hours you listened to me.

I admire Matilde Aguirre so much for the person she is; her presence in the classes honors me immensely. Maty helped this book come to life in many ways, including sponsoring a radio program called *Salud, Mente y Alma* on *La Poderosa* Radio, in Miami. Matilde was firm in her encouragement; 'write the book', she would often say, 'for many will be helped'. Matilde, I thank you for believing when I did not.

My True Teachers, as I call them, students and clients, for years have trusted the work we do; you have given me a great life, but most importantly, you have taught me so much. I thank each and every one of you.

This last year, I worked with a huge number of therapists and coaches. Too many to mention, but you each left a piece of your heart with me. You each showed me a little of what it is like to be on the "other chair." Now I feel more useful to my own clients because of each of you. Thank you, and blessings!

Finally, I believe there exists a force in the universe which is all-giving, all-loving. Perhaps that force does not need to receive gratitude or acknowledgment from me, but I assure you that its presence was strong as the words you are about to read poured out of my fingers. I am glad we are now partners.

# PART 1

# LET US GET ACQUAINTED

# 1. INTRODUCTION

Welcome to your journey. The journey you are about to embark on is very personal; you have your own reasons for taking this journey, your own motivations, and your own feelings. You are a unique individual, with unique needs and abilities. You have a unique story; only you know what you really went through, and your true capabilities. Yet, one thing is common to all of us: the need to become Awesome Again.

This program was designed for men who feel as though they are losing their edge. I did not set out to design a program like this; I simply served clients who came to the office for hypnotherapy and coaching. In time, however, compiling what was working for some men proved useful for others.

One day, I scribbled some notes, which later became the first version of this book. The first manuscript came to life, but life got in the way of publishing it. The manuscript sat on a hard drive for more than one year until I had my own crisis. Months into my recovery, I remembered this manuscript and thought that something in it could be useful to me personally. As I worked with the Steps to become Awesome Again, I casually edited the manuscript for a couple of months without much progress. Then, my good friends, Mary and Allen Vallei, invited me over to their lovely home in New Mexico for what became a mini retreat.

On the flight home from New Mexico, I did something out of character for me: I initiated a great conversation with the passenger next to me. I knew then that I was a new man. The old manuscript no longer expressed my message to you, no matter how much I edited it. So, in another move, totally unlike my previous self, I deleted it and wrote the entire book again.

The overall theme of the book, and the Steps to become Awesome Again are the same that were tried and tested during more than 20 years of clinical experience; but the writing is fresh and, hopefully, much clearer.

This program has five parts:

1. The A-test.
2. The Foundations of Awesomeness.
3. The Seven Steps.
4. The Routines of Awesomeness.
5. The guided meditations in your personal portal at www.flaviolife.com/aa.

The first part of the program is a test, but do not worry, this is not a test you can pass or fail. In fact, no one will ever know your score, only you. The "test" is simply a series of questions you will answer honestly about your present circumstances. You will then score your test yourself and learn about what your score means. The test is designed for you to overcome denial about your true situation, and for you to know that you are not alone. Many men well into their 80s and 90s, are living Awesome lives; they are healthy, sexually active, and financially stable. Yet the majority of men experience a general decline in all aspects of their lives despite living at a time of unprecedented opportunities.

Once you take the A-test, you will face the reality of where you are in terms of your potential as a man and have a good idea of where you could be. The test is very important for your overall success with this program. Do not allow a natural fear of the truth to scare you away from facing your true situation because knowing precisely where you are as you begin this program is the first step to becoming Awesome Again.

The second part of the program introduces you to the Foundations of Awesomeness and presents theoretical ideas that will open your mind up to new possibilities for you. This information is presented in a simple yet profound manner. Based on more than 20 years of clinical experience working with men who want to become Awesome Again, this part of the program is designed to open up enough space in your mind and heart so that the Seven Steps make sense and work for you.

The third part of the program is composed of Seven Steps you will take on your journey to become Awesome Again.

The fourth part of the program will help you design routines that sustain your journey into Awesomeness. You will learn to install new habits into your daily routines that make each of the Seven Steps second nature to you, a part of your daily routine. Once these Steps become a part of your new routine, you will take the A-test again and compare your score with the first time you took the test at the beginning of the program. You will notice that the quality of your life will have improved vastly.

The fifth part of the program is in your personal portal at www.flaviolife.com/aa. There, you will find the guided meditations necessary to change your mind about yourself at the level of the subconscious mind, which is necessary for permanent and smooth change, as well as many other resources that complement your experience with the program. Your personal portal will become your personal friend.

You will get maximum benefit from the program by going through each of its parts, but you can do that in several different ways, once you have taken the A-test. Some men enjoy reading the entire book once and then returning to the sections they feel they need to work on the most. Another possibility is to study in detail each section and Step before moving on to the next one. In clinical practice, we cover some of the philosophical content and aspects of each Step in each session. You can do the same with this book; you can read a chapter on the Foundations of Awesomeness and then work on a Step each time you read.

Whatever sequence works best for you, please resist the temptation to skip any part of the program, for it is designed as a complete program with each part depending on the others. If you are not sure about how to proceed, read the entire book once, and follow the suggestions and guidance in the book and in your personal portal at www.flaviolife.com/aa.

This improvement in the quality of your life is important for not only you but also all those around you who need you at your best. You may sometimes feel alone and even not needed anymore. Perhaps your children are independent or you never had any; your spouse may not be around or you never had one. Perhaps your parents left this world, or left you a long time ago. Perhaps you do not like or have any pets. You may feel that no one needs you, and feeling not needed may be a huge part of why you lost your edge.

When a man does not feel needed, he stops working on himself, for himself, and for others. When men do not work on themselves, they deteriorate, they go down fast. Yet, I am asking you to improve the quality of your life for you AND for those around you. A positive feedback loop develops when you begin to work on yourself and improve the quality of your life. As you feel better, you feel that you have more to give, and as you feel that you have more to give, you FIND people to give it to. As you become more generous, you will find that others need you and begin to rely on you. Although this may seem like a bad idea, being needed and supplying the need of others strikes at the very essence of masculinity. You will feel good serving others around you, being needed, being useful, being productive, and adding value to other people's lives. In essence, you will become Awesome Again by serving others, and that is only possible if you first serve yourself by becoming Awesome Again.

# 2. THE A-TEST

I work with men who feel that they have somehow lost their edge. Sometimes, they ask me what is happening to them, because they are not sure whether what they are experiencing is a normal part of aging or an actual problem that can be solved.

This lack of clarity causes a man to oscillate between behaviors that are really an attempt to compensate for the loss of his edge – people sometimes refer to that as a midlife crisis – and a resignation that he just is not the man he used to be. It is sad to note that each time a man goes through this cycle, he loses something else and becomes accustomed to a lower version of himself.

The A-test will help you determine where you are and what you can do to improve the quality of your life. Taking the A-test is an important aspect of your journey to become Awesome Again.

Men come to my office to deal with elevated stress, sleep difficulties, smoking, drinking, health concerns, or financial turmoil. Rarely, a man calls about his relationship; the woman usually makes that call. Few men call about the use of pornography, sexual dysfunction, or gambling. I never received a call from a man who said that he had lost his edge and wanted to become Awesome Again.

When a man takes the A-test, however, and we talk about what the results mean, they realize that the initial problem about which they called is one consequence of a larger issue that can be overcome.

There are 10 questions on the A-test. The minimum score you can possibly get on that test, if you follow the instructions, is 10 points, the maximum is 40 points. You are going to score each question from 1 to 4, then add all of them. The starting average score for the men I worked with using this process is 19 points. If you score a little lower than 19 points on the A-test, do not worry about it; it just means that we have some work to do, but you are going to be fine.

Taking the A-test is like looking into the mirror. We normally do not see ourselves as we actually are; we each tend to see ourselves through several layers of our own biases and perceptions. Just imagine what you might look like physically if you had never looked into a mirror to adjust your look. When you take the A-test, you come to see yourself more realistically, opening up the possibility for well-directed work to improve the quality of your life.

Designing a test for anything can be challenging. A test may be too sensitive and generate too many false positives, meaning that it detects what is not there, or the test may not be sensitive enough and generate too many false negatives, meaning that it does not detect what is there. A good test must also be specific enough, only catching what it is designed to catch, and not catching conditions other than what is wanted.

As an example, imagine a new test for diabetes. A good test for diabetes would detect all people who actually have the condition but none who do not have it. A good test for diabetes must also only produce a positive result for those who actually have diabetes, not other illnesses.

The design of psychological tests is a science itself. A well-validated test requires a series of comparisons between the results of a candidate test and a gold standard. The ideal test would ask all the pertinent questions and no more. You want the test to be as short as possible and yet produce the correct answer to the question it aims at answering. No test is perfect, of course, leading to the idea of a margin of error for the results a test produces.

The A-test is not a scientific test as explained above. The A-test evolved over years of work with men who came to see me for a number of problems, who expressed frustration with some sort of "loss" they could not articulate, and who wanted to be and do better.

The questions in the A-test reflect the most common issues I found working with men who wanted to be better. Men who take the A-test find it useful as a tool of self-reflection and goal setting.

In essence, the A-test reflects how you assess the quality of your life, a very subjective concept. It turns out, however, that men who score above 35 on the A-test also believe and report a very high quality of life, while those who score in the 15-20 range report a poor quality of life.

If you scored 35 or higher on the A-test, you could benefit from this program immensely by practicing the guided meditations found in your personal portal at www.flaviolife.com/aa.

## *Take The A-Test to Find Out Your A-Score*

There are ten questions in the A-test. Your answers are totally private. You can answer them on a separate piece of paper, your phone, or a tablet. Record your answers somewhere, since you will have to add the numbers to come up with a final score, and you will need this information for a later exercise.

Answer each question as quickly as possible. In other words, answer with your first impulse or thought. Do not think about the questions; just read the questions and let your fingers write the numbers.

For each question, circle or write a number, from 1 to 4. Then add all your answers below to determine your final A-score.

1. Are you now in love?
    a. No or never: 1
    b. Just a little or a long time ago: 2
    c. Somewhat or recently: 3
    d. Yes, absolutely: 4
2. Do you love someone, anyone?
    a. No way: 1
    b. Kind of: 2
    c. Yes, I think I do: 3
    d. Absolutely, with all my heart: 4
3. Do you feel healthy?

   a. No, I am very sick: 1
   b. No, but I think I am okay: 2
   c. Yes, but I have a few complaints: 3
   d. Yes, very healthy: 4

4. Do you have a satisfactory sex life?
   a. No, never: 1
   b. No, but I am okay with it: 2
   c. Kind of, but it could be better: 3
   d. Yes, absolutely: 4

5. Do you feel successful, are you in charge of anything?
   a. No, not me: 1
   b. I used to, but not anymore: 2
   c. Sometimes at work: 3
   d. Oh, yes; I decide my destiny: 4

6. Do you feel "well off" financially?
   a. No, I have debts: 1
   b. No, I barely make ends meet: 2
   c. Yes, sometimes I have a bit extra: 3
   d. Oh yes, I am proud of my wealth: 4

7. Do you have a social life?

   a. No, I am all alone: 1
   b. No, but I have one friend: 2
   c. Yes, sometimes, I get together with friends: 3
   d. Oh yes, I enjoy my social life very much: 4

8. Do you have a hobby or hobbies?
   a. No, not me: 1
   b. Well, I enjoy some things on my days off: 2
   c. Yes, I have one, but don't get to do it much: 3
   d. Yes, I enjoy my hobby(s) very much: 4

9. Are you married?
   a. Never: 1
   b. I was once: 2
   c. I am married, but the marriage needs work: 3
   d. Yes, I am married, and we love one another: 4

10. Do you happily practice any form of religion or spirituality?
    a. No, never have: 1
    b. When I was a child I did: 2
    c. Sometimes I do: 3
    d. Yes, it is an important part of my life: 4

If you are under 30 years of age add 6 points to your total.

Now add all the numbers you circled or wrote down here: __________

This is your A-score. Keep your answers and your score safe for a future exercise.

# 3. EXAMPLES OF SUCCESS

## *Meet John*

John was 52 years of age when he came to see me. John was a successful director of a large firm, yet he felt deflated. He actually kept using the word "deflated" to describe how he felt.

Our first task was to unpack the term and learn what he meant by "deflated." John was frankly obese, smoked a lot, and was in poor health. John had been married for years but claimed to feel completely alone; he actually said that he did not have a relationship with his wife. John had two children, but he did not bond with them; he told me that he barely knew his kids.

The wife and children did not "bother him much" during the weekends, which he mostly spent on his computer, basically playing, he said.

John scored 17 points on the A-test; he was not feeling very well when we met. John recognized that many years earlier he felt a lot better. He felt stronger, healthier, more successful, with hope for a better future, with some fight in him. John wanted to be Awesome Again. He wanted to get his sense of joy and zest for life back, and he wanted to get to know his wife and children.

John and I hit the ground running, we discussed every aspect of his life in detail and used hypnosis to make the changes he chose to make. John threw away his cigarettes, started to adjust his weight, and had a thorough medical evaluation. He started participating more in the family, often feeling surprised by how awesome the wife and kids were. Then it happened for John.

After a particularly productive session one Friday evening, John decided to surprise his family with breakfast the next morning. He woke up so early that the grocery store where he intended to get the supplies for breakfast was still closed. John waited in his car for the doors to open while practicing a self-hypnosis technique he learned during our sessions together. When the grocery store opened, John got out of his car.

With tears in his face, John told me that he "saw the Sun" for the first time in his life. We talked about that metaphor, but I knew exactly what John meant by "seeing the Sun." John and I worked together a little longer, mostly him marveling at how different and better his life was now. One evening, I came out of a session and found John sitting in the lobby. John was with his wife, who apparently wanted to come over and say, "Thank you."

## *Meet Luis*

Luis' mother called to see if I could help her son. Luis began smoking pot in junior high school. He quickly started experimenting with other drugs and routinely got drunk. He dropped out of high school and attended several treatment programs, some voluntarily, others mandated by the Courts. In one program, he was isolated from family and friends for 60 days.

Eventually Luis quit all hard drugs, got a GED, took a job at a restaurant, purchased a car and rented an efficiency. Luis' mother thought things were going well, until he began drinking again, crashed his car, lost his job and moved back in with mom. That is when I met Luis.

Luis was a tall and lanky 28-year-old man, quite pale I thought, for someone living in South Florida. His eyes were sunk in and dark. He did not smile. At first, I actually thought Luis had suffered bilateral Bell's Palsy, but his face was fine.

Luis clearly did not want to be at the office, he seemed to be there to do his mother a favor. Luis did not believe he *could* change, so he was not engaging; but the condition for taking him on as a client was that he would attend sessions for one week before deciding if this process was right for him.

I started describing several examples of people who had achieved "the impossible" and, quite by chance, talked about Chuck Yeager breaking the sound barrier in 1947. Luis shifted on the chair! Our daily sessions continued, and I used more aviation examples. On Thursday Luis asked me if I thought he could be an aircraft mechanic. "I would love to work on them birds" he told me.

That was when Luis committed to his own life. He never missed a session, even though he had to take two buses to get to the office. Luis used alcohol to quiet thoughts he could not manage and to sleep. Luis needed to talk his feelings out and sleep way more. We worked with each of the Seven Steps for several weeks, although I never brought up the alcohol.

Luis got a job, purchased another car and eventually rented another efficiency. One day Luis comes into the office and shows me a letter. He had been admitted to GTB technical college in Miami, where he would become an aircraft maintenance technician. We kept working together, using hypnosis to enhance each of the Seven Steps on his journey to become Awesome Again.

Luis never mentioned alcohol again. One day he came to his session with a young lady who he introduced as his girlfriend. The young lady seemed proud of her new boyfriend. Soon our work was done, Luis had become Awesome Again.

Then it happened: I opened the mailbox and found a note from Luis. He had graduated and was about to start a position at the airport "working on them birds". Luis: you are my hero!

# 4. MY OWN EXPERIENCE WITH THIS PROGRAM

I can tell you that I did not just write the book and create the program on how to become Awesome Again; I also used the program myself to get out of the tightest spot I have been in in my life.

I had been on the Mystical Path for most of my life, but when my second marriage ended, I broke apart. That profound personal breakdown led me into the darkest night of my Soul.

Many people helped me get through this ordeal, but the Seven Steps to become Awesome Again saved my life.

I will tell you what happened and how I got out of it after I tell you all about how you too can become Awesome Again.

# 5. AWESOME AGAIN FOR WOMEN

This textbook is one part of the Awesome Again Program. With the purchase of this book, you also receive access to your personal portal at www.flaviolife.com/aa where you find the guided meditations that will make it possible for you to achieve permanent change in your life.

The bulk of the textbook is composed of "The Foundations of Awesomeness, the FOA" and the actual Seven Steps you will take on your journey to become Awesome Again, the 7AA. Think of the FOA as the theory you may need to work with for your mind to help you become Awesome Again.

Becoming Awesome Again is all about changing your mind about yourself. The mind, however, sometimes resists changes until it understands why it is changing, and that it *can* change. All the information your mind may need to cooperate with you on this journey is in the FOA section.

Each of the Seven Steps is a shift in your awareness, a change in your mind, that leads you into a process, not an action or an event, but a process. These Seven processes tend to become lifelong habits for you, particularly when you use the guided meditations in your personal portal.

By far, the most common question asked about the program concerns women. Both the FOA and 7AA, the actual Steps to become Awesome Again presented here, apply equally to men and women. Women experience devastation and loss just as men do. Women also come to see me to transform their lives, usually around their peri-menopausal years.

Working with women is different from working with men because a woman's emotional constitution is different from a man's. Furthermore, the Steps a woman needs to change her life are different, and presented in a different sequence. As an example, few women need to be encouraged to Deep Talk to someone.

We have a more effective program for women to transform their lives, but I still encourage them to read this book, particularly if they have a man in their lives. Whether he is a son, a father, a brother, a friend, or a significant other, she can be helpful and support him in his transformation if she is familiar with this process.

Men, if you have a woman in your life who understands you and supports you in your transformation, you are blessed indeed. If you do not have a woman in your life right now, and if you want one, do not wait until you have her in your life to start the program. Quite the opposite, if you want a lady with you, you need to get started with this program immediately, become Awesome Again soon, and then you may have a woman with whom you both can grow together.

Many people are counting on you; they need you to be their hero. I want them to look up to you, I want the people in your life to be proud of you; I think you know what I mean by that. It is important that you restore your place as their hero.

# PART 2

# THE FOUNDATIONS OF AWESOMENESS

# 1. INTRODUCTION

This section of the book presents a good deal of information on the topics of philosophy, therapeutics, and science as they pertain to becoming Awesome Again.

The background information included in this section supports the idea that you *can* change your life and become Awesome Again. I learned many years ago, that some people do not invest the energy necessary to change their lives until they *believe* they *can* change. For some men, belief in the possibility of a better life starts with authoritative information. If you are that man, you will find enough information here to convince you that you *can* change. If you do not need all of this extra background information to invest yourself in your own journey to Awesomeness, simply skip ahead to section 3 of this book and start working with the Seven Steps immediately.

It is challenging to make this section relevant and informative to all of you. If you are a philosopher, therapist, or scientist, you will find the corresponding treatment of these topics in this book quite superficial. If you have not studied one or more of these topics before, you may find the descriptions, as presented here, somewhat challenging.

Use your own judgement to decide when you want, or need, to read this section of the book. Sections 3 and 4 of the book contain the practical Steps necessary to become Awesome Again. Section 2 contains background information that some of you may prefer to read after working with some of the Steps.

As you work with the Seven Steps to become Awesome Again you can always return here and read the sections that interest you. My suggestion to you is this: if you decide to read section 2 before working on the Seven Steps, and if you feel overwhelmed by the information presented, simply go to the Seven Steps and return to the Background section at a later time. Once you begin working on Step 6 of your journey to become Awesome Again, you may want to read more about many topics of importance to you.

Just as the Seven Steps to become Awesome Again evolved from over 20 years of clinical practice with hundreds of men, the topics presented in this section of the book are also the same ones that most men at the office discuss or ask about during their private sessions.

Men, it is time to get to work!

# 2. THE PHILOSOPHY OF AWESOMENESS

## a. What Is a Paradigm and Why Does It Matter?

A paradigm is a worldview, a way of looking at the world and, consequently, a way of looking at ourselves. If you look at a human being and see an organism, then you would address any problem that person has organically. If you see that human being as a mental entity that condenses into a physical body, then you would address problems from a mental perspective.

Here, you see illustrated two alternative ways of looking at a human being, the organic and the mental models. There are other ways of looking at humans, such as the holistic model. Each of these models is actually an entire paradigm because, according to how you see a human being, you will understand and define problems and, more importantly, come up with solutions to those problems.

The term "holistic" comes from the word "whole." The holistic paradigm does not ignore the physical. The holistic approach sees the human being as a physical, energetic, mental, and spiritual entity simultaneously.

One paradigm is not better or worse than the other. Approaching life from a holistic point of view includes having detailed work done at a physical and mental level when needed. There is nothing wrong with immersing yourself in the physical paradigm and solving physical problems through physical means. Limiting your existence to a physical phenomenon, however, will never produce the results you want.

Think of the holistic paradigm as a controller on a flight control tower observing planes flying at all altitudes. Now think of the spiritual paradigm as the pilot flying at the edge of space, the mental paradigm as the pilot at 40,000 feet, and the physical as the pilot taxing the plane on the ground. No pilot, plane, or passenger in this example is more or less important than the other; they are simply looking at different aspects of the flight, just as when we look at our lives from a spiritual, mental, or physical point of view, we are looking at different aspects of our nature. The truly holistic approach allows you to observe yourself at all levels simultaneously so that you are better able to make the appropriate change at the appropriate level needed, always considering the totality of what you are.

In order to illustrate the importance of a paradigm, consider a man who feels like he is losing his Edge, as an example. This hypothetical man is feeling sadness, lack of pleasure, not having a good time in life, not feeling successful; he has low energy, is not sleeping well, has gained weight, and feels like doing nothing all day.

If you subscribe to the organic paradigm, you would bring this man to a physician. If that physician is a psychiatrist and the man describes what he is feeling, he might receive a diagnosis of depression. If you bring that same man to an endocrinologist, who looks at the body from a different point of view, the same man might receive a diagnosis of hypothyroidism or low testosterone levels. Each of these physicians would treat that man in very different ways, but through physical means, such as medication or surgery, depending on many other details of the case.

If you subscribe to the mental paradigm, you would bring that man to a psychologist perhaps. The man may receive the same diagnosis of depression, but now the treatment may involve talking endlessly about his childhood, clearly a mental intervention.

If you subscribe to the spiritual paradigm, perhaps you would bring the same man to a spiritualist who may determine that the man has karma from a past life, for instance. The solution to the problem may involve becoming a volunteer at a shelter for the homeless, since service to others may cancel karma.

The holistic paradigm may recognize, in this example, a man with karma, who holds unresolved issues from childhood, which resulted in health problems. This man may benefit from volunteer service to the community, he may need to talk his issues out, and he may need medications to feel better sooner. Approaching the problem from all three perspectives simultaneously may expedite his healing.

This overly simplistic example illustrates the importance of a paradigm in becoming Awesome Again. How you see the world and yourself determines not only how you understand problems and objectives in your life but also what sorts of tools and solutions become available to you.

If you have been told that you have a given problem, X, which must be treated in Y fashion, know that what you have been told is simply the result of looking at life from the perspective of one paradigm. Consulting a different practitioner of the same paradigm is not truly seeking a second opinion. Becoming Awesome Again requires looking at your life from a holistic point of view and making ample use of experts in all paradigms, as the need arises.

## b. The Organic Model

As you embark on your journey to become Awesome Again, you will encounter many experts on the organic model from whom you will learn a great deal and receive services. Every man is different and is starting his journey from a different point.

Becoming Awesome Again from an organic point of view may require treating many types of conditions or diseases by different physicians, depending on where your health is at the outset of your journey. Even if you believe you are very healthy, I still suggest you have a complete medical evaluation if you have not had one in more than one year.

As a way of illustrating the organic model, it may be useful to consider the basics of four conditions that some men may have to talk to their health care provider about: depression, low testosterone, diabetes, and hypothyroidism. The discussion that follows does not in any way substitute medical care, and it certainly is not a complete description of these conditions. This section is included here simply to illustrate how, looking at an effect through the lens of a paradigm will determine the understanding of available causes and, therefore, the treatment options. As a secondary benefit of reading this section, if you are not familiar with these conditions, you will develop some good questions for your physician.

## *About Depression*

Within the confines of the organic model, depression is seen as a problem of deficiency in a neurotransmitter called serotonin.

The central nervous system, brain and spinal cord, derive its function from the function of individual cells called neurons, and from the way in which these cells are connected.

Electrical charges move within neurons. This movement can be measured as an electrical signal called an action potential. Neurons are all interconnected, but they are not connected physically. There is a little space between neurons called the synaptic cleft.

Two neurons, therefore, do not communicate by the transmission of the action potential, but by a molecule that is released by one neuron and absorbed by the other. These molecules are called neurotransmitters. There are many known neurotransmitters, serotonin being one of them.

Little vesicles inside of one neuron will open up when the action potential arrives at its end, releasing the neurotransmitter it contains into the synaptic cleft.

Serotonin can be absorbed by the next neuron from the synaptic cleft, and if enough serotonin hits it, eventually that neuron will fire as well, generating its own action potential.

The transmission of the action potential to the next neuron down the line will result in some sort of thought, action or movement, depending on the neuron involved. A neuron connected to a muscle, for instance, will release the neurotransmitter acetylcholine, causing muscular contraction. The brain, with its billions of interconnected neurons, functions as a neural network capable of the functions you are familiar with.

The idea that a lower concentration of serotonin in the synaptic clefts within certain regions of the brain causes depression goes back at least 50 years. This idea is known as the serotonin hypothesis of depression.

The serotonin hypothesis says that low serotonin levels either prevent or decrease the probability of neuronal activation, leading to a depressed mood in the individual thus affected.

If the serotonin hypothesis is correct, and some clinical evidence suggests it may be, the way to treat the depressed patient chemically would be to make more serotonin available to these neurons.

There are a few pharmacological strategies to get this done. The most common one is to prevent the reuptake, or the sequestering, of serotonin from the synaptic space by neurons. The idea is that more serotonin being available to impress upon the next neuron increases the probability that other neurons will fire, elevating patient mood. This class of medication is called a SSRI, or Selective Serotonin Reuptake Inhibitor. SSRIs bind to serotonin reuptake receptors in neurons, making the cell less likely to remove the neurotransmitter from the synaptic cleft.

For some people, SSRIs work really well, although this class of medication is also used to treat other conditions that have nothing to do with depression. Some people who use SSRIs resolve their depression in a few months and successfully discontinue the use of the agent. Other patients feel better for a while, but later report that the problem never went away.

Imagine taking caffeine to feel more energy when you have not slept well; it eventually catches up with you, and alertness is decreased no matter how much coffee you drink. Something similar seems to happen with some patients, they feel better on the medication for a while, but, eventually, their mood is depressed again. At that point, dosages are typically increased carefully. Eventually the dosage of a medication can become toxic, at which point, the class of medication used has to be switched, and the process starts again.

Some patients are eventually diagnosed with refractory depression, or treatment-resistant depression, since the condition does not respond to medication anymore. The final tool used against depression is electroshock, or electro convulsive therapy.

The progressive worsening of certain depressed patients being treated medically suggests that none of these treatment choices are addressing the cause of the problem. If the problem is not getting better, the cause is not being mitigated or eliminated. You would expect anything to get better if the cause of the problem is being addressed properly.

Many men who are now ready to become Awesome Again feel depressed and have tried medication. They tell me that they feel better for a while but eventually feel depressed all over again. Although I never suggest a man alters his medication regimen in any way without strict consultation with his physician, the cyclic improvement and deterioration of the problem, to me, suggests that the true cause of the problem is not being addressed adequately by medications alone.

You may have also arrived at the same conclusion on your path to becoming Awesome Again. You may have to do something different from now on, and although the use of medication might be a part of the overall process, you may want to do some internal work and get in touch with something deep within yourself in order to become Awesome Again.

This is a great conversation to have with your prescribing physician. Ask if there is anything other than taking medication you can do to enhance and expedite your healing if you have been diagnosed with depression.

## *About Low Testosterone*

Testosterone is the so-called male hormone, although women's bodies also produce it in lower amounts. In men, testosterone is produced mainly in the testicles. As men age, testosterone levels tend to drop. Among the many consequences of low testosterone levels are reduced muscle mass and obesity.

The combination of reduced muscle mass and obesity is critical because these two conditions feed off each other in such a way that both tend to become worse over time. First, muscle tissue consumes more energy than other types of tissue; reducing the total amount of muscle in the body also reduces the energetic consumption, predisposing the individual to weight gain. Second, the lower the muscle mass, the weaker a person feels, and the less physically active they tend to be, further predisposing the person for weight gain. Third, excess weight itself makes physical activity, such as sex, more difficult, again increasing the likelihood of further weight gain. As you can imagine, reduced testosterone levels creates a combination of factors that conspire together to make the situation worse over time; the less muscle a man has, the higher the tendency for weight gain, and the fatter a man gets, the higher the probability of accumulating more adipose tissue, fat. Lastly, fat itself makes one fatter.

There are essentially two types of "fat" in the body: subcutaneous fat, which has a yellow color, and visceral fat, which tends toward the brown color. Subcutaneous fat is fat under the skin, those are the love handles and what you pinch when you fold the skin on your belly. Underneath all that there is "bag" that holds all abdominal organs called the peritoneum. Inside this bag, within the peritoneum, is where visceral fat is found.

Visceral fat is different from subcutaneous fat in that it is metabolically active. Metabolic activity means that a tissue consumes energy and substrates (fuel), and generates byproducts, typically metabolites and heat. One enzyme found in visceral fat is aromatase, which converts testosterone into estrogens.

Visceral fat, therefore, works like a gland, producing enzymes such as aromatase which itself produces estrogens, the female hormone, from testosterone, the male hormone.

Lack of testosterone makes a man gain weight, gain fat, and lose muscle. Fat makes a man lose testosterone and produce the female hormone, which in itself generates all kinds of other problems. This is a difficult vicious cycle to break. The system becomes unstable quickly; that is why, initially, it is so difficult for an obese man to lose weight.

It is also true that weight gain, by itself, will cause reduced levels of testosterone; even when initial levels are adequate. For this reason, it is important to adjust your weight as you embark on your journey to become Awesome Again.

Many men ask me if they should just inject testosterone in order to lose fat and build muscle. My suggestion is to resist that temptation and talk to your physician about this matter. Be sure to find a doctor who specializes in hormone replacement therapy (HRT) for men. There are great doctors who specialize in HRT; they do this all day long, so their experience is invaluable.

Remember that testosterone can also activate malignant cells and have other deleterious effects when in excess or when out of balance in the body. This is one area where the expert guidance of a specialist is well worth your investment.

The good news is that there are natural ways of adjusting testosterone levels. You will find that as you go through your journey back to Awesomeness, many problems tend to resolve spontaneously for various reasons that will become clear as we proceed.

## ***About Diabetes***

Every cell in the body needs fuel to function. The prevalent cellular fuel is glucose, a form of sugar. Because it is a fairly large molecule, insoluble in the cellular membrane, glucose cannot just enter a cell at will. Most cells have special gates for glucose to enter called transporters. In order for these transporters to open and allow the glucose molecule to enter, another molecule must be present, insulin. Think of insulin as the molecule that knocks on the door, prompting the door to open, so glucose can enter the cell.

Ideally, when a cell needs fuel, insulin causes the transporter to open, allowing available extracellular glucose to enter. If the transporter no longer responds to the knock of insulin, not as much glucose can enter the cell. This is known as insulin resistance, which leads to one out of four types of diabetes known.

Only one type of diabetes concerns us here, because there is no way an adult man could have any of the other three types of diabetes and not know about it. Actually, one type of diabetes would only affect a man indirectly: gestational diabetes happens when a pregnant woman who does not have diabetes develops high blood sugar levels only during pregnancy. In the United States, conventional prenatal care includes a screen for gestational diabetes. If you know of a pregnant woman who does not have access to adequate prenatal care, do what you can to help her get it. Becoming an Awesome man includes being generous.

Another type of diabetes, less common, is diabetes insipidus. Deficiency in the pituitary hormone vasopressin, or a problem in the kidney not responding to the hormone, causes a person to excrete large amounts of urine. A person with this condition would know they have it.

Diabetes Mellitus type 1 used to be called juvenile diabetes because young children affected with this disorder would fail to thrive, unless given insulin. Insulin injections as a treatment for this disorder only became available in 1922. Frederick Banting, Charles Best, and John Macleod shared the Nobel Prize in 1923 in medicine for this amazing feat of ingenuity and creativity.

This leaves us with diabetes mellitus type 2, also known as adult onset diabetes, also known as the silent killer. DM2 is considered a lifestyle disorder because its principal cause is excess food and lack of exercise. As such, DM2 is thought to be preventable, and possibly reversible.

DM2 begins with insulin resistance. Insulin, produced by the pancreas, is available, but cells decrease their response to insulin, preventing some glucose from entering. Lower intracellular glucose levels account for the lethargy commonly associated with this disorder. If glucose is not entering cells, it accumulates in the blood initially. The body does not like too much sugar in the blood, so it saves the excess as fat.

A common response to the cyclical lethargy associated with DM2 is hunger. People thus affected tend to eat snacks, worsening the problem. Many people are affected with this disorder, or a precursor to the disorder, and do not know about it. A person with constantly elevated blood glucose levels is prone to increased glycation, partly responsible for the hardening of small blood vessels, which causes many unfortunate consequences.

During the precursor stage of DM2, called pre-diabetes, or simply insulin resistance, a person would experience wide variations in blood glucose levels. This wide variation has medical consequences, but it also creates an emotional rollercoaster for the affected person that can seem brutally cruel. A man who has pre-diabetes may not know about it, and, certainly, he would feel like he is losing his edge.

The good news is that a very simple blood test in the morning can detect this condition, and its effects are reversible with drastic lifestyle changes.

## *About Hypothyroidism*

The thyroid is a gland at the base of the neck that has a lot to do with metabolism. For various reasons, sometimes, the gland becomes hypoactive, meaning that it is working below normal levels.

A person affected with hypothyroidism would experience a general depression of all functions in the body. The person would be less active, and, most likely, feel cold. The skin, nails, and hair would be dry. The person may feel depressed and a little sluggish; they typically gain weight.

A man may be affected with hypothyroidism and not know about it, at least, if the condition is marginal or not severe. This man would feel that he is losing his edge, that he is getting old, and that he no longer has it, when, in reality, he needs a thorough medical evaluation, and adequate care. Once the exact physical problem is known and treated, that man can look for other means of possibly ameliorating his condition.

Not all blood exams check thyroid hormones automatically. If you suspect you may have a thyroid condition, please ask your health care provider for an examination and specific blood tests sometimes referred to as "thyroid panel."

## c. The Mental and Holistic Models

You read about some answers the organic model might produce for the man who wants to become Awesome Again. The above was only a very brief overview of the way a paradigm works, not a review of the medical literature, much less medical advice. Still, I hope it is evident to you now that, even a person who subscribes to the holistic paradigm, can, and should, benefit from expert medical care.

In order to illustrate the mental model, let's return to the same hypothetical man described earlier, who is feeling sadness, lack of pleasure, not having a good time in life, not feeling successful, has low energy, is not sleeping well, has gained weight, and feels like doing nothing all day.

A strict mentalist would say, "What you're feeling is all in your mind. Don't worry. Just change your mind, think positive thoughts, and everything will happen for you; you'll be Awesome Again."

The truth is that the strict mental model has been tried and found not to be quite so effective. People begin to think positive, start to act, and proclaim things such as "Fake it until you make it." Many people have been faking for a while and they have not made it. Eventually, people abandon the ideas that do not produce the intended results.

I propose looking at things differently and using the Holistic Paradigm. Look at the whole human being, for when you do, there is no question that there is something about us that is physical. Beyond the physical aspect, there are thoughts, that is, the mental aspect. Beyond the physical and mental, there is something else. If we stripped a man of his body and mind, would he still exist?

Even without a body and a mind we still exist. Some names for what is beyond body and mind are spirit, soul, consciousness, heart, or emotions. People are free to use whatever word for what is left if body and mind are no longer there, but most agree that something remains. Here, we are going to call that something else beyond body and mind a "soul," but do not get too hung up on terminology for now.

It is important to look at life holistically because, as you are going to read about, every effect has many types of causes. One has to do with the reason why something happens. Often, until we learn and remedy the reason, that something cannot change. When a man wants to be Awesome Again, the loss of his edge has many levels of causes that must be addressed.

When we look at life from these four perspectives, physical, energetic, mental, and spiritual, we are looking at the whole human being, hence the term "holistic."

We learned about the physical or organic model. We learned about the mental model and the holistic model. We are not just physical beings. Sometimes, truly solving a problem requires looking at all four dimensions in which we exist. A problem that exists only in the physical dimension should have a physical solution. When no physical intervention makes an apparently physical problem go away, the problem cannot be physical only.

## d. Physical Problems Are Real

Having learned about different paradigms, the organic, mental, and holistic models, keep in mind that the mental and holistic models do not deny the veracity of the organic model. In other words, when we look at the human being holistically, and talk about spiritual and mental factors to life, we are not denying what scientists who work on the organic model have discovered.

The issue here is one of causation; what truly constitutes the cause of a problem? The holistic model claims that organic findings are not the cause but the consequence of something that comes before that.

Thoughts, particularly if intense and sustained over time, tend to produce an organic response, for instance. The organic response is real but is the consequence of a thought. The thought itself may be the consequence of a prior cause, such as the achievement of a spiritual purpose in the person's life. Treating only the physical body, therefore, without realizing the higher purpose for the problem, would only result in temporary amelioration, with a likely resurgence of the problem in a different form. Consider this example:

The acupuncturist at the office and I once worked with a person so heavy that we could not use the treatment table we had. The man told us that he weighed close to 400 pounds, but we could not measure his weight because the scale we had only went to 300 pounds. This man had been treated with appetite suppressants for most of his adult life, losing weight each time but gaining it right back, and more, once he discontinued the medication. In deep hypnosis, he talked about a previous life in which he was very unhappy. That life ended by suicide. In this lifetime, he always felt tempted to kill himself for no apparent reason. He felt that by weighing his body down he would anchor himself to the Earth, and "not go." If the story ended here, most people would find his imagination wild and continue looking for the right medication or surgery that would finally make him lose weight permanently.

Our sessions became more existential and philosophical, even mystical at times. He and I never discussed his weight or his body, but he started to change. The last time I saw him, he was visibly happy; and he had lost 70 pounds with no diet or medication.

In this example, you see how the physical problem of obesity was caused not by lack of appetite suppressants, but by a series of thoughts, most of which the person was not even aware of. The thoughts were the result of a strong decision made before he was born. His spiritual self had a very clear purpose for this lifetime: to overcome the temptation to kill himself. In his case, overcoming the temptation to kill himself required being in a situation where he would consider that suicide would be "justifiable" somehow, given how hopeless his problem was.

In this example, what was the cause of the obesity? Clearly one must overeat to become obese, but what causes overeating? Overeating resulted from a thought "I must anchor myself to the Earth." That thought resulted from a spiritual decision to overcome the temptation to end his life prematurely. In the past, when he would treat the problem only chemically, the problem would decrease for a while but come back worse each time. Since then, I have worked with dozens of people who had bariatric surgery and regained weight. They have all told me, "They operated on my belly, but what I really needed was surgery in my mind."

Saying that organic findings are not the cause of the problem in no way means that we should not treat the physical body when needed. Treating the body promptly and adequately is important first because the person is suffering, and secondly because, in some cases, without urgent physical intervention, they may die.

The true application of the holistic model does not deny the importance of treating the body through physical means; quite the opposite, the body should be treated according to the holistic model. If only the body is treated, however, and there is no change at a higher level, mentally and spiritually, the physical problem tends to become chronic.

## e. What Is Cause?

In philosophy, the concept of causation or causality is very important. I once presented a paper at a conference on causality. I started the talk saying that a person had the common cold because the price of gas had gone up. The word "because" establishes my claim that the cause of the person's cold is the increase in the price of gas. I explained that the common cold is caused by the rhinovirus. The rhinovirus creates symptoms when immune function is compromised. Immune function is compromised by increased stress. Stress levels are elevated in times of economic hardship. An increase in the price of gas creates economic hardship, thus the common cold was caused by the increase in the price of gas.

This satirical introduction was meant to introduce two ideas. One is that many levels of causation exist; therefore, it is not always possible to establish one cause to each effect. Secondly, a domain shift occurred in the causation chain. The first two causes, the virus and depressed immune function are physical, but the stress produced by economic hardship is a mental phenomenon. In this example, one level of causation is more immediate than the other but not truer.

Probably the first philosopher to discuss causation was Aristotle (384-322 BC) who lived mostly in Greece. Aristotle denounced the singular notion of causation, as in A causes B. Aristotle claimed that there are four different levels of causation that must be considered for any effect: the material cause, the efficient cause, the formal cause, and the final cause.

Aristotle uses the example of a marble statue to explain his theory of causation. The actual marble is the material cause of the statue, for if there were no marble, there would be no marble statue. But marble alone does not a statue make. Somebody has to do something to the raw marble in order to transform it into a statue; that is the efficient cause of the statue. The sculptor imparts a form to the raw marble in order to transform it into a statue; that is the formal cause. Finally, the whole process has a purpose; that is the final cause.

David Hume (1711-1776), another philosopher, claimed that there is no such thing as cause. What you and I call cause is just a habit of the mind, Hume would say. When two events occur reliably together, the mind tends to call one the cause, and the other the effect or consequence. The first event observed is labeled by the mind as cause, and the second as effect. According to this view, if every time a switch on the wall is pressed, the light goes on, the mind will conclude that one causes the other. Pressing the switch on the wall becomes the cause of the light going on, but, according to Hume, it is not so. The mind links two separate events, calling one the cause and the other a consequence. David Hume is known in philosophy as a skeptic.

Immanuel Kant (1724-1804) contributed to the issue of causation with an eloquent response to Hume's arguments, and philosophers still debate whether or not there is cause, or if a cause can be known. Modern philosophers talk about going back to the Aristotelian tradition of multiple causes. Various theories suggest different layers of causation such as necessary causes, sufficient causes, and contributory causes. Establishing that A causes B is not always easy, yet, from the perspective of the holistic model, the spiritual domain causes what happens at the level of the mind. What happens at the level of the mind causes what happens at the level of physicality.

Later, you will learn about *how* the mind affects the body because it does. The body affects the mind as well, but physical experiences that affect the mind are themselves, in some way, generated by the mind. Much of what happens mentally serves a higher purpose, a spiritual purpose. The spiritual dimension, therefore, is seen as the cause of the mental. As an example, consider a person whose *spiritual purpose* in this life is to become humbler. This person may think negatively, leading to a physical illness. Disease can create pain, which puts the person in a bad mood. Here you see how a mental phenomenon (negative thinking) created a physical result (disease), and how the physical result itself changed mood, a mental phenomenon. In other words, mind changed the body, and the body changed the mind. Furthermore, the physical illness, in this example, humbles the person, thus achieving the original spiritual purpose.

Ultimately, all physical findings serve a spiritual purpose, which is equivalent, in Aristotelian terms, to saying that the spiritual is the ultimate cause of the physical. This notion of causality does not deny the veracity of what happens in the body, and it does not mean that we should not treat the body. What it does mean is that neglecting the mental and spiritual aspects of any problem only invites it to morph into another problem, eventually becoming worse.

This discussion may seem a little dry, and perhaps even irrelevant, but it is not. The discussion of causation is intended to release you from the exclusive adoption of the physical paradigm, as though it were the only reality that exists. To become Awesome Again, you have to look at the whole person that you are. Consider your mind, your thoughts, including the ones you are not conscious of, and your emotions. Consider the connection between you and the universe, which is your spirituality. The resources in your personal portal at www.flaviolife.com/aa will help you *feel* this connection. If you do that, you are well on your way to becoming Awesome Again.

# 3. THE THERAPEUTICS OF AWESOMENESS

## a. Mind, Systems and Thoughts

Becoming Awesome Again requires a change in your mind. Specifically, you will change your mind about yourself. Changing your mind entails an understanding of whether the mind exists, what it is, how it creates your reality, how it affects the body, and how it operates; in other words, we have to learn what we are dealing with in order to change it.

### *Is There Such Thing As "Mind"?*

Some people are surprised by the question: "Does the mind exist?" because they assume that everyone agrees that it does. However, there is a long tradition of thinkers and experts who would claim that there is no such thing as the mind. Experts, such as Dr. Sidney Walker, a psychiatrist, would claim, "There is no 'mind' without the brain" in his 1997 book *A Dose of Sanity*.

In your personal portal at www.flaviolife.com/aa, you will find other resources and references that will help you decide for yourself if there is such thing as mind. There, you will also find a powerful paper arguing for the existence of the mind, since, for the purpose of this book, we assume that the mind does exist. This book proposes becoming Awesome Again by changing your mind about yourself, and that which does not exist cannot be changed.

## *Okay, It Exists, But What Is Mind?*

The Merriam-Webster dictionary defines "mind" as "the part of an individual that feels, perceives, thinks, wills and especially reasons." The dictionary does not define mind, it describes some of its functions and activities. Although we all know what we mean by "mind," it is simply not easy to define it accurately.

A strict philosophical definition of "mind" is beyond the scope of this book. It may be useful, however, to think of "mind" as an interface between the spiritual and physical aspects of a human being. Using a modern computer as an analogy, the mind would be the software, including the operating system, that runs the various programs.

If the software/operating systems analogy seems useful to you, think of the mind as such a sophisticated system that it reaches self-awareness, just as computers and robots do in science-fiction movies.

It is important to note that the mind is not who or what we are. Who and what we are uses the mind to achieve its purposes in the world, but it is not the mind.

According to the Kyballion, which contains the Hermetic philosophy of Ancient Egypt and Greece, a hypothetically perfect mind would produce a perfect life, since a human life is a reflection of a spiritual ideal, the reflecting plane being the mental. Since few lives on the Earth are perfect, few minds are perfect.

## *Mental Systems*

Since we cannot quite define the mind, let us describe it, and some of its functions, via an analogy with the physical body.

The physical organism is understood in terms of several systems with different functions, such as the cardiovascular, the digestive, the nervous system, and others. Think of the mind as a mental organism, the mental body, with several different systems, just like the physical organism.

The physical system most closely associated with the mind is the nervous system. The nervous system has a sensory and a motor aspect. It functions as a storage device and makes decisions, such as in reflex actions, without mental involvement. Finally, the nervous system creates, as in the cellular proliferation, regeneration, synaptic remodeling, and myelination, ideas that will be made clear in the *neuroplasticity* section of the book.

The mind also has a sensory and a motor aspect. A part of the mind perceives what is happening, and another part of the mind plans and executes actions. The mind also has a storage aspect, as in memory, and an intelligence aspect, which is the ability to reach a conclusion from several premises. Finally, the most mysterious aspect of the mind is the creative; the mind creates what we perceive as our reality.

Sensory, executive, storage, intelligence, and creative are the five systems within what we call the mind. Understanding that mind is actually an organism with several systems clarifies why there has been so much historical disagreement regarding the existence and description of the mind.

To complete the analogy between the physical and mental organisms, consider two more ideas: First, just as cells are the units of life throughout the physical body, thoughts are the units of life within the mental body. Secondly, just as the physical body has an external aspect and an internal, hidden, aspect, so does the mental body. We refer to the external, visible, aspect of the mind as the conscious mind, and the internal, hidden, aspect as the unconscious.

## *Origin of Thoughts*

All cells in the physical body come from one cell, called a zygote, formed at the moment of conception when the male sperm enters the female egg. The egg itself is one cell, and the sperm deposits its share of chromosomes into the egg, giving us our 46 chromosomes, or 23 pairs. The zygote divides and differentiates, eventually making about 100 trillion cells that compose an adult human body.

The zygote, therefore, is the ultimate origin of all physical cells, but a given cell in an adult human body may have one of three immediate progenitors: The mother cell such as in the epidermis and the dermis, the source such as the bone marrow, or an external source such as in a viable implant of some sort.

Now consider that thoughts are to the mental body what cells are to the physical body. Thoughts are units of life within the mental body just as cells are units of life within the physical body.

A given thought can have one of three origins. A thought may originate in the source such as in the soul; we call that an inspiration. A thought may originate in the environment such as in sensorial perception. Finally, thoughts may be produced by the mind itself as combinations of other thoughts such as in what has been called the reactive mind. Metaphorically, we could say that thoughts can come from "above," from "below," or from "within" the mind itself.

Thoughts from "above," or inspirations are unmistakable. They are brief but intense; they change your mood and often lead to immediate action. Thoughts from "below," the awareness of sensorial perception, are similar in that they are also brief. You might catch yourself thinking *This room is cold*; that thought is your awareness of a sensorial perception. Both of these types of thoughts can persist in the mind and combine with one another, producing offspring. The sum total of those thoughts that originated in the mind itself has been called the "reactive" mind because it always produces a reaction, not an action. Reactive thoughts include words like "and," "because," or "besides," such as in the phrase "The table is white because John doesn't like red."

John may not like red, and the table may be white, but the causal connection between the two is a thought generated by the mind itself. The soul did not make that connection, and senses cannot inform you of it.

As you can now tell, a great deal of mental activity is reactive. Reactive thoughts consume a lot of energy and constantly produce new offspring, such as in "The table is white because John doesn't like red, because he's cheap."

Just as a physical cell consumes energy, creates a product, and reproduces itself, thoughts do the same. From a therapeutic point of view, when we look for "the cause" of a persisting negative or detrimental thought, we are looking for the parent thought. Finding and healing the parent thought is important because each parent thought may have many offspring thoughts.

Offspring thoughts are combinations of other thoughts, some from above, some from below, some from within. When a person is "con-fused" (think with fusion) they are experiencing the fusion of many thoughts together, some of which can be contradictory, leading to the sensation of paralysis.

This is important because thoughts lead to feelings and actions. Actions determine results in life. On your journey to become Awesome Again, you will encounter many thoughts that no longer serve you; it is time to discard many old thoughts. The thoughts that must be discarded, the ones causing the problem, cannot be the inspiration or the sensorial perception, they must be the reactive thoughts, produced by the mind itself.

There are two ways to eliminate unwanted thoughts; one is by focusing your attention only on the inspiration and on the sensorial perception. When you notice a reactive thought, immediately observe something objective, such as the size of the tree, the color of the sky, the height of the building. Later, you can still the mind and listen for inspiration. When the mind is focused on the task immediately in front of you in the present moment, there is no room for reactive thoughts. By always focusing your mind on a task, you are effectively eliminating reactive thoughts.

The second way of eliminating unwanted thoughts is the analytical route. When you observe a reactive thought intruding into your awareness, ask yourself, "Where is this coming from?" You will soon recognize that you became aware of an offspring thought and found one parent. But reactive thoughts have two progenitors, just as people have two biological parents. The mind combines two thoughts to form a third. The analytical route can be laborious, but, sometimes, it is necessary to find these progenitor thoughts because a correction, such as forgiveness, may be in order.

The notion that each reactive thought has two progenitors that combine, eventually creating a problem is important therapeutically because each effect must be preceded by two causes, not one. This explains why some people report the return of a problem after "the cause" was eliminated. People say, "I went to a therapist, I found this out, and the problem went away for a while, but it came back." This happens because one of the causes remained active and eventually partnered with a new thought to produce yet another offspring. The parent thought reproduced itself again; from the perspective of the person, the problem goes away for a while and comes back later.

The mind is essentially a tool that allows the spiritual to interface with the physical. As a tool, the mind can be impressed by the soul, by the information obtained from the physical senses, and by itself, through the conclusions, judgements and ideas it generates based on other thoughts.

Changing your mind about yourself in order to become Awesome Again is largely about eliminating reactive thoughts that were never "true" to begin with. Sadly, we suffer a great deal because of thoughts our own minds make up.

## *Conscious and Unconscious Mind*

The difficulties associated with defining and describing "mind" notwithstanding, if someone were to ask you several questions, I suppose you would agree that your answers would emanate from your mind, indicating that we all have a working understanding of what mind is, even if we cannot define it.

If you keep asking a person about themselves, you will come to a point beyond which they will no longer be able to answer. This point is referred to as the limit of conscious awareness. All of the material the person hypothetically has access to and is capable of expressing would comprise the conscious mental content. Beyond what a person is consciously aware of in terms of information, motivations, and intentions, there is more material. Because the person is not aware of that content, it is referred to as "unconscious" or "subconscious." Some schools of thought define the unconscious as all that we are not aware of, but recognize that some of that content has to do with the individual only, the subconscious, while a larger bulk of the unconscious is collective, the supraconscious or, as Carl Gustav Jung (1875 – 1961) called it, the collective unconscious. Technically, therefore, the subconscious is a portion of the unconscious, but for our purpose here, these two terms will be used interchangeably because they both refer to the portion of us that we are not aware of.

Hypnotists typically credit the unconscious with functions such as long-term memory, running autonomic bodily functions, and self-preservation. This last function implies protecting the person from threats, real or perceived.

Mystics would agree with the above functions of the unconscious, but they would add one more: The unconscious is responsible for creating the circumstances that allow the purpose of a life to manifest and be experienced by the person. This means that if the purpose for that lifetime is for the person to become humbler, for instance, the unconscious will find the most effective means of achieving that result. If the best way to instill humility is through adversity, the person will experience adversity, all created by their own mind but unconsciously. The conscious mind may be aware of the adversity, but may be unaware that it was created endogenously.

Mind was defined as the interface between the physical and the spiritual worlds. Different systems within the mind are processing information originating in the physical world and originating the means to satisfy physical needs. Other mental systems attend to the purpose for this lifetime and ensure that the person creates, albeit unconsciously, the circumstances necessary to live that purpose.

The two faces of the mind, conscious and unconscious, occur in every mental system. The mental body is composed of a sensory, executive, storage, intelligence, and creative systems. As a spiritual entity living a physical existence, we are only partially aware of each of these systems and functions. The so-called conscious mind is the extent to which we are aware of these functional systems. However, we remain unaware of the greater portion of each functional mental system; that portion is what we call the unconscious mind.

One functional mental system is the sensory, our ability to sense or perceive information from our surroundings. Many kinds of studies show that our awareness of our surrounding is extremely limited; furthermore, that awareness is highly specialized and variable through training. As an example, a private citizen may not notice two men talking at a corner as he drives by. The police cadet may notice the men talking. The experienced police officer may notice that one of the men was an undercover police officer, and the other a suspect of interest to the police. Sensory perception increases with training, but it is also specific to the interest of the person. The experienced police officer may not have noticed the scent of freshly baked bread coming from the same corner, for instance, because he was focused on the men talking.

The hypnotic state allows the person to become consciously aware of the unconscious. In this example, the experienced officer may not remember any particular scents in that corner, but in the hypnotic state, he may be impressed by the vividness of the olfactory impression registered.

The conscious/unconscious dichotomy applies to all functional mental systems. A person does things that they are not aware of, such as involuntary actions and behaviors. Conscious memory is extremely limited and selective. Decisions can be utterly devoid of reason, in which case, we rationalize prior behaviors. And most strikingly, we create our own circumstances, even those that we do not want or like.

On your way to become Awesome Again, you are going to become aware of the part of you that you have been unconscious of, and you will use that awareness to create an Awesome life. This is how you make true, effective, long-lasting changes in your life. In your personal portal at www.flaviolife.com/aa, you will find guided meditations specifically designed and created to help you become more aware of your unconscious existence.

## b. Why It Is Difficult to Experience Mental Causation

*If you have faith the size of a grain of mustard, you can move a mountain.*

*—Jesus*

You know that the Earth revolves around the Sun, but if you did not know it and simply looked at the sky each day, what would you say about the movement of the Sun? This is a loaded question because it presupposes the answer, the movement of the sun. Our senses inform us that the Sun moves, not the Earth. You can sit on one chair, perfectly still all day, and observe that the Sun comes up on one side of the sky and goes down the other. Your observation would warrant the conclusion that, because you never moved, the Sun must have. But in this case, the senses are deceived, for the Sun did not move, you actually did.

If I were to tell you that your mind creates your own reality, you would nod in agreement because you can remember a few times when things happened in accordance with your wishes. But if we examine painful and frustrating memories, those that you really dislike in your life, it would be very difficult to conclude that your mind created them, just as it is difficult to conclude that you moved, not the Sun.

Sometimes we embrace the idea of mental creation, but at other times, we shun it. When it comes to disease, for instance, we tell ourselves that "things just happen, no one knows why." The medical establishment reinforces this notion in order to function. When it comes to wealth, however, truly wealthy people, not those who temporarily have money as a result of winning it, all tell you that they became wealthy in their minds first, then in their bank accounts.

From the perspective of the person, just as in the moving Sun example, it is difficult to experience mental creation or causation. This difficulty can become so extreme in some cases, that some people simply remove the mind from the creation equation. These people would subscribe to the idea that "it is all about working hard," as if hard work is not, itself, the product of a mental process.

A given physical result in your life can manifest through one of four mental pathways or, more commonly, through a combination of two or more of these four. Suppose you wish to eat an apple pie. You can go get it yourself, you can get someone to get it for you, you can intuitively walk into a store that is giving away apple pies, or you can cause the apple pie to manifest out of thin air. These are the ways your mind creates physical results:

1. Direct action: hard work.
2. Personal influence over others: management.
3. Organic circumstances: luck.
4. Manifestation: magic or miracle.

No matter what strategy or combination thereof was used, all physical results started as an idea, a mental phenomenon. The person may be aware of the idea or they may be unaware of it, reflecting the possible unconscious cause of mental creation.

You may like some results you created in your life, whether you created them consciously or unconsciously. But you may suffer a great deal and dislike other aspects of your life that you are now ready to change, to create something better in its place.

We all started our lives being trained in direct action to achieve desired results. You worked hard to learn to walk, read, and write. You were told to work hard in sports and school. You were told to get a job to get what you wanted. Direct action was the first strategy you learned to get results in early life; therefore, it is the strategy you default to when you have a problem later in life.

When you first wanted to regain your edge, you worked hard on this. You went to the gym, you ate less, and you dressed up for a while. Some of you purchased a sports car, others found a girlfriend; some did both. Those watching you said you were facing a midlife crisis, but you pressed on, saying that this is the new you. You used direct action to achieve a desired result; you felt better for a while, but ultimately you gave up on your efforts because they did not work, meaning they did not produce the intended result, or the intended result did not last. Some of you had given up on yourselves until you found this book.

Because most men have given up on themselves, or are close to giving up, by the time they find this book, there is a natural resistance to the notion of mental creation as presented here. Men tell me, "I tried that; it doesn't work for me. Just tell me what to do, not how to think!"

These men are having a hard time experiencing mental creation, or causation.

Temporal proximity between any input and an output gives the mind the certainty of causation. If you press a switch on the wall and a light immediately turn on, you think of pressing the switch as the cause of the light going on. If the light took two weeks to turn on after you pressed the switch, you would have a hard time concluding that the operation of that switch is the cause of the light.

Take exercise and weight loss for instance. Exercise causes weight loss. Studies show however, that the longer a person fails to lose weight while exercising, the more likely they are to quit, while knowing fully well that exercise causes weight loss.

If a person consumes a toxin and experiences pleasure, they will conclude that the cause of the pleasure is the toxin. That person may continue to consume the toxin, seeking pleasure. The toxin may cause all kinds of pain and even death, while the person seeks more of the toxin, thinking of it as the only way to experience the original pleasure.

As you read the two examples of causality above, hopefully you are thinking that the explanations are incomplete, for there are other causes at work in each case. The person who exercised and did not experience weight loss may have eaten more, for instance. The person who consumed the toxin felt pleasure because his brain released certain chemicals that create the sensation of pleasure. These brain chemicals, neurotransmitters, can be released without consuming the toxin, and the toxin causes other unwanted side effects that are not pleasant.

This is a very important idea for you to become Awesome Again: the resultant cause. For the sake of this example, allow me to oversimplify the issue of weight loss. There are two causes, not one cause, of weight loss: exercise and caloric intake. What actually causes weight changes in this simplified version is not one or the other, but the balance of the two. The balance of the two, exercise and intake, is the resultant cause of weight loss or gain.

A resultant cause has a magnitude and a direction. The expressed intention may be to lose weight, but the resultant cause may be in the opposite direction.

The weaker a resultant cause is, the longer it will take for the effect to manifest physically. The longer it takes an effect to manifest, the less likely one portion of the mind is to accept the creation of another.

It is difficult to experience mental causation because of temporal separation between cause and effect. Temporal separation is inversely proportional to the magnitude of the resultant cause. A stronger resultant cause will generate a physical effect or consequence sooner, reinforcing the notion of mental causation to that person. A weaker resultant cause will delay the physical manifestation, decreasing the person's belief in mental causation.

When a man tells me that he is doing everything right, yet it is not going his way, I must examine more deeply what he claims to want to create, on one hand, and what else he is doing that may be taking away from his intended results, decreasing the magnitude, or reversing the direction, of the resultant cause on the other hand.

The notion of a resultant cause includes both conscious and unconscious causes. As an example, consider a man who is struggling financially. He states the desire to create wealth, he works hard, he improves his ability to manage others, he reads books on positive thinking to improve his luck, and he prays to win the lottery. This man is setting in motion all four levels of causation discussed above, but he is still struggling financially. Unconsciously, this man may believe that "money is dirty," or that "rich people are dishonest," for instance. That unconscious belief may be so strong in that man that it literally changes the direction of the resultant cause he wishes to manifest.

Unless this man addressed the unconscious beliefs that affect this resultant cause, he would not experience financial freedom any time soon. In time, he would deny mental causation and lose the motivation to win.

When I say that it is not happening because the resultant cause is not strong enough, some men tell me that it may not be happening because they started off too far behind. After all, they would say, it would take longer to lose 100 pounds than it would to lose 10 pounds.

We call this the illusion of distance between desire and result. The illusion of distance is only real insofar as it is one more cause that goes into the resultant. There is no distance effect; no one is ahead or behind. Besides, some men have lost 100 pounds much faster than others have lost 10 or even 1. Your belief that you are starting off too far behind is one cause that pulls you in the opposite direction you now claim to wish. Let go of the illusion that you are "behind" in your life. Focus instead on the desired result and work on aligning each aspect of your life in a coherent direction that strengthens the resultant mental cause.

There is a special guided meditation in your personal portal at www.flaviolife.com/aa that will help you achieve a higher state of coherence, increasing the magnitude of the resultant cause in the direction you want to go with your life.

## c. Changing Your Mind About Yourself

I help people change their minds about themselves so they can succeed by becoming who they really are. If we only look to the world outside of us and our reactions to it as the source of our own vitality, we are going to be depleted quite quickly because the world is of a negative polarity as compared to the human essence. The human essence, being divine, is of a positive polarity in relation to the world it inhabits.

As human persons, we "live" between the divine and the world. The divine is positive; it charges us. The world is negative; it depletes us. We receive from the divine; we give to the world. We are free to choose our source of energy, our source of inspiration. The ideal situation would be to live in the world, to make a contribution to the world, without being depleted. This is only possible when we are being recharged by an Infinite source. If you look at people who try to attain any type of satisfaction and inspiration from the world, they all become exhausted and depleted quite quickly.

What does it mean to "plug in to an infinite source of inspiration"? Think of a human being as being composed of a body, mind, and soul. The soul is already divine, inhabiting the divine. Not much can change at that level. In Kabbalah, they refer to that aspect of our existence as Neshama, a stable source of Life.

The physical body must function within the laws of nature. The body itself is not very different from that of other higher mammals, thus being guided by similar instincts. The body functions within very narrow operational limits. Every physical, environmental, and physiological parameter we can think of and measure must be kept close to the optimum if disease or death is to be averted. Just think of temperature, as a simple example. How much variation in temperature can we really tolerate? A few degrees each way, before we freeze or become heat exhausted. Yes, we can use intelligence through technology to alter the proximal environment, such as in heating or cooling the space we occupy. But still, if we are to operate effectively and stay alive, the artificial microclimate we create must not deviate too far from the optimum.

Plugging into an infinite source, therefore, must mean a change in the mind. "Changing our minds about ourselves" means to reorient the mind to look within as our own source of inspiration and vitality. Once we learn to do that, everything else begins to flow. This reorientation of the mind is equivalent to the chiropractor turning on innate flow or the acupuncturist turning on the flow of chi. In other words, by plugging into an infinite source, we have infinite vitality available to us.

The first step needed to change your mind about yourself in the way just described, is to remove blockages to the natural flow of vitality. Anthony de Mello said that when the eyes are unobstructed, the natural result is vision. I learned that when the mind is unobstructed, the natural result is vitality.

Blockages prevent us from looking into our own source because they become the focus of our attention. Think of addiction to alcohol for instance. The toxicity of the alcohol prevents much of a connection between physical and soul. In fact, alcohol is an anesthetic and an amnestic. How can a man remember who he really is while ingesting large quantities of a powerful amnestic? How can a man feel what he must feel to evolve while ingesting large quantities of a powerful anesthetic? Right, he cannot. But that is not his worst problem. His worst problem is his primary focus. What does the mind of the addict focus on all the time?

Correct, the object of his addiction, whatever it is; in this example, it is alcohol. His mind is actually focused on the very thing that is robbing him of his life all the time. The mind drives us toward what we focus on, which means that, unless we change our minds about ourselves, addictions tend to get worse over time. We must change our minds about ourselves in order to become Awesome Again.

Any substance or behavior that robs you of your vitality becomes the focus of your attention, driving you deeper into the problem itself. Men are built and wired to solve problems, fight enemies, overcome problems. Men are made to focus on the immediate problem in front of them exclusively. We have a narrow, sharp focus, and we don't like to lose our vitality. Loss of vitality means no hunting, no game, and death. So, that which robs us of our vitality becomes front and center; we focus on it more and more to the point of obsessing.

You will become Awesome Again by quitting all toxic substances and behaviors, including overworking, lack of sleep, pornography and gambling.

We need to discuss one more thing. This is much more difficult for men to talk about than the use of toxic substances, although this is usually the root of all other problems. This will block and prevent the connection with the higher aspects of ourselves. I am talking about emotional trauma, and the typical resentment and anger that follows. Consider three types of anger and ask yourself if any of these apply to you.

The first type of anger is the explosive type. This is exemplified in the man whom everybody identifies as the angry one, who is always shouting, screaming, beating people up, breaking things. A1 is the easy type of anger to identify. This man could be very nice most of the time, but as soon as some trigger is activated, he blows up. That is the A1 man.

The second type of anger happens when a man is super quiet, never says anything mean to anyone, but, inside, he is burning up with frustration and anger. That is a huge problem because this quiet man will eventually blow up. He can blow up outwardly, like the quiet man who one day picks up a machine gun and kills a bunch of people, or he can blow up inwardly, as in the man who suddenly drops dead from a heart attack or drops out of the window of a 40-story building "accidently." A2 is an angry man, but that man has many emotional barriers to get through before we can talk about anger.

The third type of anger is the guy who says, "No, everything is fine; I'm not angry," but everybody around him is basically blowing up and fuming in anger. A3 instills anger in others through a number of well-placed injustices, false promises, and contradictions. A3 is usually a very intelligent man who knows how to turn things around. People around him always feel blamed and inadequate. A true A3 would not be reading this book unless life totally broke him down, all the way down. If that is your situation, we have a lot of work to do, but you are not alone.

Toxic substances and emotional blocks must be removed in order to become Awesome Again. Daily meditation is a great way to begin the process, and a good amount of hypnosis or self-hypnosis will install the habit of daily meditation for life so you can be Awesome Again. If anger is your challenge, remember that in your personal portal at www.flaviolife.com/aa, you will find other resources specifically directed at helping you release your anger. All resources found in your personal portal are free to you; they are one expression of my gratitude to you for purchasing this book.

As a parting thought, think of the mind as a parabolic dish that picks up satellite signals. The dish could be oriented to one satellite or another. Think of one satellite in this analogy as the physical world and the reactive mind, and the other as your own spiritual world. This has nothing to do with religion, but everything to do with the higher aspects of your own being. In meditation, we are reorienting the antenna; rather than looking to the outside or to the reactions, we begin to look toward our own source, our own light within.

Hypnosis is a great way to instill a habit, specifically the habit of meditating daily. The true effects of meditation are felt when it is practiced daily. Meditation only takes a few minutes, but those few minutes invested in yourself will pay big dividends. The highest return on your time investment on your way to becoming Awesome Again is in practicing a few minutes of true meditation each day.

If all of the above seems like a lot of material to digest, please do not worry. This section is only meant as a broad overview of where we are going together. Later, we are going to discuss specific steps you will take to become Awesome Again.

### d. All True Change Involves the Subconscious Mind

Think of the many things you do all the time that require no thought. When a person walks, there is a huge amount of muscular and nervous coordination taking place to keep us going and to not fall down. We typically refer to that as "walking" or "balance," but it is a very intricate and complex task. Each of the muscles involved in walking can be contracted at will voluntarily, but we do not think of contracting and relaxing each muscle in sequence when we walk; we simply walk. From our point of view, the coordination that allows all of the biomechanical operations that result in walking are organized by the subconscious mind. We do not have to think about it. We think of the outcome, such as, *I'm going to the kitchen for a glass of water,* and the subconscious mind coordinates all of the muscular contractions and relaxations necessary to get us there and back. Speaking of water, digestion is another example of subconscious coordination.

You can think of many examples of things you do all the time without thought or attention. It is possible to carry out these actions without thought because they have been programmed into your subconscious mind as a routine that runs automatically. The benefit of running a routine from the subconscious mind is that it frees the rational mind for something more immediate or urgent. So, when we walk, by not having to think of each step, we can carry out a conversation, for instance.

Everything we do without thinking is mediated by the subconscious mind. All habits fall into the category of things we do without thinking. Some habits are good for us, such as brushing teeth; others may not be good, such as being disorderly.

Everything you identify as something you now want to change is an acquired habit. If you want to start getting up earlier in the morning, you are saying that you got in the habit of getting up late, and now you want to change that habit. Since all habits are programs running in the subconscious mind, it follows that all true change involves making changes at the level of the subconscious mind first.

The subconscious mind does not have values; it does not judge the orders it receives as good or bad, for instance. The job of the subconscious mind is simply to execute the orders that have been loaded into it. In principle, any desired change can occur by simply loading a new order into the executive portion of the subconscious mind. Analyzing why the previous order was there, where it came from, or whose fault it is, is not necessary for change. The only thing necessary for change is to load a new order into the subconscious mind.

In order to load a new order into the subconscious mind, to be executed later as a new, desired habit, you need two things:

1. Learn to open the door between conscious and subconscious.
2. Learn the language of the subconscious mind.

Opening the door between the two aspects of the mind, conscious and subconscious, is as simple as relaxing the physical and mental bodies. Professional hypnotherapists are trained to use many sophisticated ways of helping other people do that. But, in essence, you can use self-hypnosis, which involves learning to relax and focusing your mind on a desired outcome, using the language of the subconscious.

The subconscious mind speaks in symbolic language. In order to load a new order into your subconscious mind, you need to find an active and emotional image that represents to you your desired goal having already been accomplished. For a person who wants to lose weight, for instance, a popular image is running on the beach, or wearing a special suit at an important party. As you use the meditations found in your personal portal at www.flaviolife.com/aa, you will learn more about loading images with emotions into your subconscious mind as a way of creating new habits.

Knowing something is not enough for that something to happen or for a man to change and become Awesome Again. As an example, I am reminded of a house I lived in at one time that required extensive remodeling in order to remove the odor of cigarette smoke. Even the air conditioning ducts had to be replaced because no amount of cleaning removed the peculiar odor left behind by the heavy and constant smoking that happened in that house. The interesting thing is that the previous occupant of that house was a lung surgeon. That man knew something about the effects of smoking on the lungs, yet he smoked quite a bit each night when he got home from the operating room.

Please learn how to make yourself Awesome Again by studying these pages, but know that all effective change happens at the level of the subconscious mind. That is why when you purchased this book, you received exclusive access to your personal portal at www.flaviolife.com/aa, which contains, among many other useful resources, several guided meditations specially prepared for you to become Awesome Again. Each of these guided meditations will have a profound transformative effect upon your subconscious mind. You will confirm how, within 90 days of starting this program, you will feel Awesome Again.

## e. Meditation and Self-Hypnosis

Think of meditation as the reorientation of your attention to the higher aspect of your being. Normally, your attention is focused on the outer world, and the information you acquire from it through the five senses. When you meditate, you simply learn to focus your attention on the inner self, your inner world.

The rational mind is not well equipped to focus its attention on the inner world. The subconscious mind does that job well. By definition, none of us are rationally aware of our subconscious minds. It follows then, that the rational mind becomes aware of the subconscious, while the subconscious mind is already tuned into the inner self. That first step, when the rational mind becomes aware of the subconscious, is called hypnosis. If you are doing this by yourself, it is called it self-hypnosis.

When an experienced meditator meditates, these two processes happen so continuously that it may be difficult to distinguish between the two. One strategy to learn to meditate, however, is to first learn to enter the hypnotic state by yourself, then expand from there into the universe within.

Here is what you can expect to happen in your life as you learn to meditate. As you read the following list, however, keep in mind that you will realize many other benefits that derive from these presented here.

1. Your health can categorically, most definitely, improve, and your weight can be adjusted. You are going to sleep better. Everything about your health, every parameter that can be measured, can improve. This has been researched vastly and it is absolutely known that your health can improve in every single aspect. It doesn't

mean that everything that is going on in your health is going to go away magically; I'm saying that it can improve. Whatever is going on in your body can improve to a certain extent because other factors may or may not be changeable.

2. The feeling of aggression will leave your system. Not all people start off with aggression within. Those who have aggression will be free of it once they have been meditating for a while. As with all conditions in life, aggression also has a hidden face; it is called victimhood. Aggression may manifest as outward anger or as the inward feeling of being victimized. The man may feel victimized by the world, the government, other people, or even himself. The extent to which you feel like a victim is the extent to which you are also an aggressor. Socially, we may not see overly victimized people as aggressors, we tend to feel sorry for them, but these are two faces of the same coin.

3. You will feel a renewed sense of hope, vitality, and purpose. People who meditate will tell you that they feel a strong sense of purpose in life. Most men who feel that they have lost their edge, feel purposeless. Living with a sense of hope for an even better life, vitality, as in being really alive, and purpose, is simply Awesome.

4. People who have been meditating for a while feel a profound sense of prosperity not only in financial terms but also in every sense of the word. Financial prosperity will come to you perhaps by desiring fewer things, being more productive, or a combination of both. But there is more to prosperity than healthy finances; there is social, intellectual, and vocational prosperity. The term

"prosperity" comes from the Latin *pro* and *spere*, meaning "according to your hopes." In other words, living a prosperous life means living the life of your dreams.

5. Above all, your heart opens up when you meditate. I know this might be a little bit too mystical for some of you right now, but, in time, if you meditate, you are going to see your heart opening up. You will know that your heart is open because you feel connected with everyone and everything. The most wonderful feeling you can experience is feeling connected to everyone and everything. You begin to see life as one huge common thing. We are all in this together: nature, the planet, the universe. We are all part of one big thing. This feeling of unity is like being in love, but constantly and with everyone and everything; that is what I mean by opening up your heart. All of this is yours if you will take the time to learn to meditate.

There are many ways of learning to meditate. The simplest is to use guided meditations, such as the ones you have on your personal portal at www.flaviolife.com/aa, and letting your subconscious mind guide you into deeper states of awareness. Guided meditations typically achieve their effect by helping you relax mind and body and focus your attention on your breathing, while other suggestions create the intended effect.

A man who uses guided meditation daily for 30 days, about 20 minutes each day, can learn and develop the skill of meditation and derive great benefit from it.

A faster way into meditation is to use professional hypnosis. A professional hypnotist skilled in meditation can hypnotize a man and help him meditate deeply in a matter of days.

I cannot comment on or suggest the use of any chemical substances, herbal preparations, or drugs to enhance meditations because I have never used any of these adjuvants. I also come from a mystical background that sees the use of any substance for meditation as unnecessary.

True meditation can bring many benefits into your life, as described above and is relatively simple to learn. However, all people who truly meditate have crossed a threshold, they have all faced a monster that caused many to turn away and never come back. Carl Gustav Jung (1875-1961) called that side of us we have to face in order to meditate, the shadow. None of us like to face it, but until we do and learn to love it, we are a slave to it.

The notion that life only happens from birth to death is a myth. This myth excuses us from having to deal with our own distant memories and actions. Getting into meditation is difficult for some people because there are things about themselves that they do not want to remember. Yet, life is eternal. We live always and we have experiences that predate birth itself.

Also, when no one is watching, we sometimes act on certain proclivities that cause a strange mixture in us: pleasure and total degradation. The sum total of those proclivities, plus the memories we cannot easily face, constitute the shadow that prevents us from meditating deeper, like a sentinel, standing at the gates of paradise with flaming swords.

Each meditator must discover for himself that the sentinel is but an illusion, for only love is real.

# 4. THE SCIENCE OF AWESOMENESS

*Mind is the builder, physical is the result.*
*—Edgard Cayce*

## a. How the Mind Affects the Body

Philosophers have debated for centuries regarding the possibility that the mind affects the body. The problem is that the mind seems so different from the body that it is difficult to see how one could actually change the other. This debate presupposes the existence of what we call "mind," but another group of philosophers would argue that there is no such thing as mind to begin with, rendering, to them, the mind-body debate absolutely moot.

Dualists acknowledge the existence of two types of substances that are radically different from one another: the mind and the body. Monists, those who believe there is only one substance in the universe, see both the mind and the body as a continuum of possible expressions of some universal substance that is neither, in itself, mind or body.

A notorious dualist of major historical importance was Rene Descartes (1596 – 1650), a French philosopher and mathematician. In his writings, Descartes makes it clear that two such different things, such as body and mind, could not interact, but eventually settles on the pineal gland as a possible point of contact between both. Because of Descartes' historical importance and prominence, the idea that mind and body could not interact gained scientific popularity, reaching the 20th century as an accepted truth, despite a long history of the alternative view.

The two pathways through which the mind affects the body presented here are simple to understand. As you read about the mind-body effect, keep in mind that all physical changes start at the mind, as Edgar Cayce (1877-1945) so eloquently explained. This means that what your life is like today, in all respects, is ultimately a creation of your mind. This last claim is very difficult to accept, but accepting responsibility for what we have created puts us in the driver seat of our destiny, making it possible to be Awesome Again.

To be clear, if a person learns about "positive thinking," or the "law of attraction" and wins the lottery, for instance, they would accept mental creation quite readily. But when a typical person experiences something quite unpleasant to them, a common response is to label that experience as an "injustice" and fight it, instead of remedying the cause that brought it about in the first place. This behavioral response would indicate a low commitment to the notion of mental creation, making the next win less likely.

## *The Two Pathways of Mind-Body Effect*

The first pathway through which the mind affects the body is the sum total of our behaviors. If a man eats when he is not hungry, and he does that consistently, his body will gain weight. In eating when not hungry, there is planning and execution of a behavior, clearly a mental phenomenon. The consequence of that behavior will be a change in the form of his body, a physical result. Whatever the ultimate reason for eating when not hungry, the execution of the behavior is a mental phenomenon. The result, in this example, is visible physically.

A client may sometimes claim that they are not aware that they are overeating, especially when not hungry. We call this behavior mindless eating. But awareness, or lack thereof, of the mental planning and execution of a behavior does not change its fundamental mental nature.

I once saw the great Zig Ziglar (1926 – 2012) speak. He said that, for many years, he was overweight by choice. He emphasized his "choice" to be overweight as he explained that nobody had ever forced food down his throat. Mr. Ziglar actually said that each thing he ever ate was the result of a choice of his, clearly a mental phenomenon.

Overeating, which originates in the mind, and the consequent physical result of obesity is just one simple example of how the mind affects the body through behaviors. Whether a man thinks that he can avoid a behavior or not, or whether he thinks he is capable of doing something or not, does not change the fact that all behaviors originate in the mind and have a physical consequence. Now think of the millions of behaviors we engage in each day, and how we are each shaping our reality and bodies accordingly.

Addictive and mindless behaviors, such as overeating in the example above would seem to suggest an origin other than in the mind. The very word used "mind-less" confirms that suggestion, potentially creating confusion. It turns out that there are two aspects to the mind: the one we are aware of, by definition, is the conscious. The one we are not aware of is, again by definition, the unconscious. Two clarifications are in order here:

1. The notion that there is a part of our minds of which we are NOT aware has been firmly established, both by the original psychoanalysts about 100 years ago, and by modern scientists, specially neuroeconomists. Beyond what science can inform us about ourselves, any man who has searched for a motivation for doing or not doing something, any man who ever asked himself, "Why did I do that?," acknowledges the existence of a part of himself he is not aware of.

2. The terms "unconscious" and "subconscious" are being used here interchangeably, but technically, the unconscious has an individual portion called the subconscious and a collective portion called the supraconscious.

If the mind affects the body, and if bodies are detrimentally affected all the time, as in dis-ease, it would mean that the mind is creating dis-ease and even death. But if the prime directive of every organism is to survive, how can any mind ever produce a behavior that turns out to be detrimental to the organism? It turns out that all detrimental behavior is mediated by the subconscious portion of the mind. This explains why no amount of talking, or asking a person why they do something detrimental to their health will ever yield a positive change. The subconscious motivation for the behavior must be elicited and transmuted into something positive for the individual.

The subconscious mind also affects the physical body through the energetic body.

## *The Second Pathway*

A central theme in Oriental medicine is the notion that there is a network of meridians and channels though which energy flows. This network of channels amounts to a double of the physical body, as each cell in the physical body is served by this energy called chi, ki, prana, vital energy, vital force, etc.

Practitioners of oriental therapeutic modalities such as Reiki, acupuncture, or acupressure would claim that disease in the physical body forms when the flow of this nonphysical energy is disturbed. This energy has different polarities; too much or too little of either polarity can create an imbalance that, if sustained over time, will manifest as physical illness.

This nonphysical energy, along with the channels though which it runs, forms an energetic matrix (think of a mold) later filled with physical cells that differentiate and assemble into specific tissues, organs, and systems, according to the "instructions" received from the energetic matrix.

In the section about epigenetics in this book, you will read about how an individual mature cell comes to look as it does and do what it does because of selective gene expression. Basically, all cells in the body come from the same single cell formed at the time of conception, called zygote. That single cell contained the entire set of genes the body will ever have, about 30 thousand genes is the current understanding. As the zygote undergoes mitosis, exact copies of the original are made. After a few rounds of division, something absolutely amazing happens: differentiation. The daughter cell, even though it has all the same genes the mother cell has, expresses some genes and not others. Selective gene expression accounts for the differences among mature cells. Roughly, it is estimated that all mature cells express about 15 thousand, out of the total 30 thousand genes. About 8 thousand genes have to do with the life of the cell, these are the ubiquitous genes expressed in every cell. The other 7 thousand genes, out of the remaining 22 thousand, are what gives an individual cell its specific form and function.

As the embryo begins to take shape, stem cells that find themselves in the cephalic end, where the head will be, express genes that turn them into eventual cephalic cells, such as neurons, for instance. Other cells find themselves in the caudal end of the embryo, where the "tail" will be, and express genes that turn them into caudal cells, potentially a Leydig cell. What causes a stem cell to express one set of genes, as opposed to another, giving it the form and function it eventually adopts, is the energetic environment it is in, the energetic matrix.

Robert O. Becker (1923 - 2008) did fascinating research, mostly with lizards and rats, showing that cells would differentiate and form tissues corresponding to the location in the body they were implanted. Nowadays, the notion that you can implant a nondifferentiated cell (stem cell) into an organ and have it differentiate into the exact cell the organ needs is commonplace. The stem cell gets instructions to differentiate selectively from the energetic environment it is placed into.

David Daniel Palmer (1845 -1913), the founder of chiropractic, and Bartlett Joshua Palmer (1881 – 1961), his son, known as the developer of chiropractic, are credited with writing the *Green Books,* in which the philosophy and practice of chiropractic is articulated.

The actual practice of chiropractic is all about locating and removing subluxations. A luxation is a joint dislocation; a subluxation would be a minor joint dislocation.

Subluxations are important because they block, at least partially, the flow of innate, the same energy Orientalists have been describing for thousands of years, but with a different name. According to chiropractic theory, the alteration in the flow of innate energy causes any form of disease or dysfunction in the physical body.

The *Green Books* explain what causes subluxations: mechanical, chemical, and emotional trauma. Mechanical trauma includes impact, falls, or being hit by a car. That would dislocate many joints. Chemical trauma includes smoking, toxic substances, excessive drinking, a poor diet, and breathing contaminated air. Emotional trauma includes strong emotions, such as anger, sadness, bitterness, rage, and others like it. The tension and stress that accompanies these emotions is certainly capable of moving bones out of position. In this case, the subluxation is created both through behaviors, such as accidents precipitated by the inattention that accompanies anger, and by the sustained physical tension or inactivity created by certain strong emotions.

Once joints of the spine become misaligned, a slight spinal nerve impingement would decrease the flow of innate down that channel, creating dysfunction or disease in the affected part of the body. Looking at a physical effect, such as a diseased organ, and tracing back to the cause of the dysfunction, we find the subluxation itself caused by an emotion or behavior of mental nature.

Chiropractic, therefore, is an accepted form of Occidental mind-body medicine, just as acupuncture is an accepted form of Oriental mind-body medicine. Both medical modalities recognize, at their core, the existence of the energetic body. The mind affects the body through the energetic body.

The energetic body has also been called the etheric body, the vital body, the quantum body, the etheric double, and other equivalent names. The energetic body is not physical or mental in nature, although it affects both, as an intermediary between them.

If the topic of mind-body medicine is important to you, a number of important resources and references are available to you in your personal portal at www.flaviolife.com/aa. For now, it is important that you know that the mind affects the body because changing your body on your way to becoming Awesome Again begins by changing your mind about yourself.

## b. A Bit About Neuroplasticity

### *Introduction*

A material can undergo elastic or plastic changes in shape. Take a common metal paper clip, for instance. Bend it slightly. When you leave it alone, the paper clip will return to its original shape. While you applied a force to the paper clip in this example, it suffered an *elastic* change in shape. Now take the same paperclip and bend it into an "L" shape. When you leave it alone this time, the paper clip retains a shape that is different from the original, even when the force you applied was removed. In this case the paper clip suffered a *plastic* change.

In engineering, an elastic change in any system is one that returns that system to its original condition when the stimulus is removed. A plastic change results in permanent change to the system, even when the stimulus is removed.

When you run up a flight of stairs once, your entire cardiovascular system experiences an elastic change, for several minutes later, the system will function indistinguishably from how it did before you climbed the stairs. But when an athlete trains every day, after months and years of intense training, the cardiovascular system will look very different from the way it did prior to the training. That cardiovascular system changed plastically.

All parts of the body experience both elastic and plastic changes throughout the life cycle. Normal growth and aging are examples of plastic changes. Filling and emptying the stomach through the ingestion, digestion, and elimination of one meal, is an example of elastic changes to the stomach.

The brain of the adult does not look like the brain of the newborn, and it does not look like the brain of that same person at the age of 90. The changes observed in that brain are examples of plastic changes, *neuroplasticity* by definition.

The big deal about neuroplasticity, as discussed since the second half of the twentieth century, is a matter of timescale. Everyone knew that the brain changes on a time scale of the lifespan of the individual, but scientists thought that on a time scale of a few years, the brain did not change much. When changes in brain structure were confirmed in multi month or multiyear time scale, as a response to function or injury, it changed how we understand the nervous system and life itself.

I want you to know, beyond a shadow of a doubt, that anything that can be measured can be improved. This is really important to helping you become Awesome Again, because you will experience many changes during the next several years. It is up to you to make these changes happen in the right direction.

Some men need more details before accepting an idea. For those of you who want more facts about neuroplasticity in order to be convinced that you can become Awesome Again, this section can serve as a good introduction. In your personal portal at www.flaviolife.com/aa, you will find a number of references to more complete sources of information about neuroplasticity.

## *Neurons and Brains*

The functional cells of the nervous system are called *neurons,* although other cells, such as glial cells that were once thought to only support neuronal function, are now thought of possibly being functionally active as well. Brain function results not only from neuronal function, but equally important, is the way in which these neurons are connected among themselves. A functional brain is therefore a *neural network*.

The connection between two neurons happens at the *synapse*, where a chemical called a *neurotransmitter* jumps from one neuron and affects its neighbor. That tiny space across which the neurotransmitter travels is called the *synaptic cleft*.

Neurotransmitters from many neighboring neurons are received by a given neuron. All of that input is integrated, and at the body of a given neuron, a "decision" is made to pass that signal on to the next neuron or not, depending mostly on the strength of the sum of inputs received.

Between the body of the neuron and its end, where it connects with another neuron, there is a long part of the cell called an *axon.* The axon is wrapped in an insulating substance called *myelin.* The thicker this myelin sheath is, the faster a signal is conducted through a neuron, and the more likely it is to be passed along to the next neuron.

On a timescale of months, changes in the nervous system, neuroplasticity, result from responses to brain injury, and from function, or lack thereof.

## *Examples of Neuroplasticity*

1. *Neurogenesis,* the birth of new neurons, is one example of neuroplasticity. You may have heard that you don't get new brain cells; if one cell dies, you have one fewer. Scientists now tell us that we do, in fact, get new brain cells. Plenty of neurogenesis happens in the embryo, but neurogenesis happens in the adult mammalian brain as well, particularly in the *hippocampus,* the *olfactory bulb* and the *cerebellum,* but possibly in other areas as well. The hippocampus is involved in memory consolidation, the olfactory bulb in odor perception and processing, and the cerebellum has much to do with the coordination of muscular contractions.

2. *Myelination,* the deposition of a thicker myelin sheath around neuronal axons, allows for a faster and more effective conduction of signals along nerve fibers, the axons. The more a neural pathway is excited, the more myelin tends to be deposited along those fibers, strengthening the likelihood that a pathway will respond more effectively in the future. If you look at a slice of brain tissue, you will see two regions: the white matter and the grey matter. White matter is mostly the myelin around axons in the brain and spinal cord, and the grey matter is mostly cell bodies, neuronal soma. The proportion of grey to white matter in the brain can change as more or less myelin is deposited around axons. This type of neuroplasticity is probably the only one that can be observed at a gross level, with the naked eye.

3. When the *action potential,* the electrical signal that travels within the axon, reaches the end of the neuron, it opens a vesicle that releases a neurotransmitter into the synaptic cleft. The neurotransmitter molecule may be picked up by a close neuron, and depending on the overall strength of the signal received by the downstream neuron, it may or may not propagate the action potential. If the probability of a signal being transmitted is increased, it is said that the synapse was strengthened. The synapse may also be weakened, a fortunate outcome when a behavior is no longer desired. Changes in synaptic strength change brain function plastically.

4. Regardless of the total stimulus received by a neuron, it may not propagate the action potential if it is not

excitable enough. *Neuronal excitability* can change, changing brain function.

5. If a signal pathway in the nervous system, particularly in the brain, is interrupted, as a result of brain injury for instance, the signal can travel through a different route and produce the same result. At the brain level, this is called *cortical remapping*. When a person does not have the use of one sense, such as sight, other senses, such as hearing and olfaction, become more acute. This is one example of cortical remapping. If you are a man who experienced a traumatic brain injury, for instance, just trust that you are not limited to what you have been told you lost. Scientists are learning more each day about neuroplasticity. Most likely, with the appropriate exercises, you can regain much function.

During your journey to become Awesome Again, you may have moments when:

1. You feel stuck in old patterns of behavior, thoughts, and feelings.
2. You cannot stop doing what you no longer want to do.
3. You cannot do what you want to do.
4. You think that being Awesome Again is for other men, but not for you.
5. You feel that you lost your edge for good.

During those difficult moments, remember these words: neurogenesis, myelination, synaptic strengthening, neuronal excitability, and cortical remapping. Just know that your entire nervous system can change if you use it in the Awesome ways we are going to cover in the Seven Steps. Yes, you too can become Awesome Again.

## c. A Bit About Epigenetics

### *Introduction*

You may be encouraged by the notion that you can become Awesome Again as you read this book, only to lose hope all over again when you talk to a person who says, "It's all in your genes, and genes don't change."

You may have heard that there is not much you can do about becoming Awesome Again because your genes determine your destiny, and, according to this view, you may be genetically predisposed to a mediocre life. Some well-intended people may even refer to genetics as an infallible science, sentencing you to a life that certainly cannot be improved.

While it is true that our genes determine much of what happens in the body, as the science of genetics explains, it is also true that a gene can only do what it does if it is expressed. The science that explains factors that may alter gene expression is called epigenetics.

This section is important to you, as a man who wants to become Awesome Again, because you need to know that you can change your body by changing your mind. This is not just positive thinking hype; this is what scientists teach us. When you combine what you learned about neuroplasticity with what you will learn about epigenetics, you will be encouraged to know that you definitely can become Awesome Again. By changing your mind about yourself, you can change your body, literally.

In order to understand a bit about what epigenetics has to do with becoming Awesome Again, it is useful to first understand a bit about genetics. This description is very short because this book is not about genetics or epigenetics. In your personal portal at www.flaviolife.com/aa, you will find a well-referenced article on epigenetics that will expand your horizons on this topic if you are new to it.

## *Genetics in a Nutshell*

The history of genetics, only about 150 years old, is a fascinating account of human creativity, ingenuity, persistence, and even luck. Geneticists first discovered what kind of substance was responsible for the transmission of information from parent to child. It turned out to be *nucleic acids*, not *proteins* as had been postulated. By 1952, the nucleic acid of interest was identified as *deoxyribonucleic acid*, DNA for short, and by 1953, the three-dimensional structure of the molecule, the famous double helix, was described.

> *Just imagine, as an exercise, a string of pearls spaced apart. Now imagine another string next to it. The pearls next to each other, but on opposite strings connect. You now picture a ladder in your mind. The poles of the ladder are the original strings, and the rungs on the ladder are the connections between every two adjacent pearls. Now take*

*this entire ladder and twist it into a spiral; that is what DNA looks like.*

Inside of the cell, that entire double helix is itself wrapped around a protein core called *histones*. The entire package, DNA plus histones, forms the *chromosome*, of which humans have 46. One set of 23 chromosomes is derived from the maternal gamete, the egg; the other set comes from the paternal gamete, the sperm.

The "pearls" we just imagined are called *nucleotide bases*, or just bases for short. In intact DNA, just as in the ladder, bases on opposite strands of the DNA connect, forming *base-pairs*. Human DNA adds up to about 3 billion base-pairs.

There are four types of nucleotide bases found in DNA, and their specific sequence can be used to convey information just as "1s" and "0s" can be used to convey digital information, or the 26 letters of the alphabet can be used to convey meaning through words and sentences. This information, much like a blueprint from which a house can be built, will be used to build proteins, which serve as the building blocks of the body, and as *enzymes* that make all kinds of biochemical reactions possible.

A number of highly specialized proteins are involved in a process known as *transcription*; that is when the DNA molecule is unwound, split apart, and copied into a new molecule called *ribonucleic acid*. This molecule carries information, by virtue of its nucleotide sequence, outside the nucleus of the cell; for this reason, it is called *messenger ribonucleic acid*, or mRNA.

Just outside the nucleus of the cell, in or around another organelle called *endoplasmic reticulum* (ER), another protein complex called a *ribosome* assembles the building blocks of proteins, called *polypeptides*, based on the information carried by the mRNA. This second process is called *translation*. Proteins are molecules built by connecting together many amino acids (there are 20 amino acids in total) and folding the resulting "string" into complex shapes. A polypeptide is a sequence of many amino acids that does not form a fully functional protein.

Proteins are important because the whole body is built out of them, and because every biochemical reaction depends on proteins called *enzymes*. The *normal* look and function of the body, therefore, depends on the sequence of nucleotide bases stored in the DNA molecule.

Just as a word is any sequence of letters that conveys meaning, a *gene* is any sequence of nucleotide bases on the DNA molecule that can be transcribed and translated into a polypeptide (protein precursor). It may be useful to think of a gene as any sequence of bases that performs a function, a definition that makes it clear why it is so difficult to know exactly how many genes there are. Imagine 3 billion letters, and how many words and phrases can be made if you transpose letters, eliminate segments of letters, and splice several segments of letters any way you want.

Out of the 3 billion nucleotide bases on human DNA, scientists have identified *roughly* 30 thousand genes. It would be tempting to think that, on the average, each gene is composed of 100 thousand nucleotide bases, but this is not the case. After mRNA is made based on the DNA (transcription) it is highly modified before it is ready to serve as a template from which polypeptides can be made (translated). Many segments of DNA do not appear to encode mRNA, and many segments of mRNA are disposed of during *modification* prior to translation. The result is that only an estimated 2% of the DNA molecule codes for actual genes.

Gene expression is the creation of a functional protein from a piece of DNA. If we think of a gene as a set of instructions, as the blueprint, then expressing the gene is like building the house. The gene product, a polypeptide, would be the house in this analogy. This means that having a gene for a particular trait or condition does not mean actually having that condition. The gene would have to *be expressed* in order for that condition to develop. This makes genetics a *probabilistic* science, as opposed to a *deterministic* one, leading to the notion of *selective gene expression*.

Out of the roughly 30 thousand genes in the human genome, just about 8 thousand are expressed in all mature cells; these are *ubiquitous* genes. In total, mature cells express from 11 to 15 thousand genes, primarily because of a phenomenon called *cellular differentiation*. When biological life first begins, all embryonic cells are similar, with the same genes expressed. At some point during development, however, as cells continue to divide to increase the size and functions of the baby-to-be, they begin to adopt specific functions and shapes. The result is that liver cells look and function differently from cardiac cells, for instance, because different sets of genes in each are expressed.

A number of genes are known to be expressed only when their products are needed by the cell. The most basic example of this phenomenon is the *lac operon* cluster of genes in *E.coli* bacteria. These genes code for enzymes needed for the metabolism of lactose. If lactose is not available to the bacterium, synthesizing the enzymes would not make sense, thus the genes would not be expressed. When the organism detects lactose in its environment, the genes are activated, expressed, and the enzymes are manufactured, making it possible for the bacterium to utilize lactose as a food source.

Human cells are different from bacterial cells in a number of important ways; they are even more capable of selectively controlling gene expression through a myriad of mechanisms. As a result of selective gene expression or repression, an entire life can be changed, one cell at a time.

## *Epigenetics and Your Health*

Too much of anything in the body is as detrimental as too little of that thing. As an example, you want the genes that encode for the hormone testosterone to be expressed, so that testosterone is made available to your body. But too much testosterone can also cause malignant cell proliferation, for instance. You do not want that.

There are genes that, when expressed, prevent disease; you want those genes expressed. There are genes that, if expressed, create disease; you do not want those genes expressed. Awesome health, therefore, depends on selective gene expression. By selectively expressing or repressing genes, cells determine not only what products are available to the body, but also how much.

The science that studies what factors outside of a cell allow it to selectively express a gene is called *epigenetics*.

We have seen one example of epigenetics already in the case of E. coli bacteria that live in the human gut. Another simple example is found in the beta cells of the human pancreas, which synthetize insulin when they detect elevated glucose levels. The synthesis of insulin requires gene expression. A change in diet changes the environment cells are exposed to, in some cases, changing what genes are expressed or repressed.

Mental attitude has been known to alter the body over the years, not only in terms of what diseases it may predispose a person to, but also in terms of the general development and shape of the body it produces.

Scientists have now confirmed that mental attitude and specific mental exercises, such as meditation and self-hypnosis, can also alter gene expression in thousands of genes implicated in disease and its prevention. Dr. Herbert Benson, from Harvard University, summarizes much of this research in his 2011 book *The Relaxation Revolution*.

As you continue on your journey to become Awesome Again, just know, beyond any doubt, that your body will remodel itself, not only in ways you are familiar with, such as in weight adjustment and muscular mass, but also at a genetic level. By adopting the Awesome attitude, you will learn about in the Seven Steps section, you will be well on your way to building a better body, and an Awesome life.

### d. Unplugging from the Source Causes Depletion

When I was a kid, my parents owned a travel trailer. Vacations were awesome because we could go places where there were no hotels; I thoroughly enjoyed, and still do, deep immersion in nature.

That trailer had different power sources: an internal battery pack, propane for the stove and refrigerator, and land power or car power.

The idea, when in a campground, was to plug the trailer into a power outlet to keep the internal battery charged and have more lights and hot water available. It was usually my job to lower the levelling jacks and bring out the extension cords each time we parked.

Looking back, it is amazing that we could function in that trailer for several days in the wilderness away from land power. The ammonia-cycle refrigerator and the stove ran on propane; the 30lbs of liquid propane we carried would probably last at least 30 days. The internal battery pack, primitive by today's standards, would keep minimum lights on for a few nights, but you could run the car's engine and recharge the battery. The battery controller would keep lights on at a constant level as the battery discharged, then shut lights off when the battery reached a low level of charge.

One night the trailer was plugged into the outlet, the lights were on, and we were playing cards. Suddenly, it all went dark. My father, recognizing what had happened, immediately rearmed the circuit breaker and the lights went back on.

Unbeknownst to us, the circuit breaker between the trailer and the incoming power had opened up. We thought we were plugged into a vast source of power, but we were running on internal battery power. For a while, we could not tell the difference between battery power and land power because the lights were just as bright, until the internal battery was depleted; then it all went dark.

So it is with a man. When a man is young, so much power is available to him that he cannot tell the difference between being connected to a source versus running on internal power. For most young men, his energy is all he needs. But, as the years wear on, just as in the travel trailer example, if a man is not connected to a higher source of power, he will eventually feel depleted and his light dims down. The man feels that he lost his edge; he is deflated, beat, depressed, sad, down, blue, and many other names and descriptions, all equivalent to the travel trailer example. That man was disconnected from his own source, most of the time, not even knowing it. The only true solution to this man's loss of luster is to reconnect to an infinite source of power.

When at the office, in private consultation, some men look at me with a smirk at this point. I can almost hear their thoughts, saying, *I knew he was going to push his religion on me.* It turns out that the infinite source of power you need to plug into may include religion for some of you but, actually, has nothing to do with it.

Think of the day before you went on a much-anticipated vacation. How did you feel? Did you get a lot done? Think of the last time you went on a date with a woman you thought was awesome. How did you feel? What about the day you got an awesome car? A motorcycle? The day you put all 12 bullets into the center of the target on the shooting range? How did you feel? That feeling had nothing to do with religion, although it has everything to do with divinity.

Sure, some men find their divinity through religion; this is one possibility. But the "active ingredient" that changes a man's life is not religion, it is the encounter with the divine within himself. That encounter begins with a change in his mind.

Depletion, burn out, or exhaustion happens when a man only nourishes his mind with thoughts from outside of himself. If a man disconnects himself from his inner nature, his inner self, his higher purpose, he will function well for a while, just as the internal battery of the travel trailer will provide illumination for a while. Eventually, however, that man will feel that he lost his edge. When he is ready to become Awesome Again, he needs to learn to look up, to seek higher thoughts, to expand his horizons, and plug into something bigger than himself, but that mysteriously is within himself.

In order to become Awesome Again, you need to change your mind about yourself enough for you to see yourself as part of something big and powerful. When you feel that you are a part of something big and powerful, you will also see that this something is always on your side, always ready to benefit you in every way. This something is benevolent and friendly. This something is the Universe.

It is actually possible to tap into the same power source that creates stars and galaxies. In fact, you are the product of a miracle yourself. What made your body possible is as much of a miracle as the birth of a star in the universe. Some men are "looking down," thinking that because the circumstances of their conception were not ideal, their lives are doomed somehow. The circumstances of your conception or upbringing do not matter. What matters is that you are here now and that you are the creator of your own destiny. Pay attention to the biological miracle that made your body possible, instead of what you were told about the conception. Plug into the miracle that makes it possible for a seed to produce a tree; for a tree to produce a fruit, and the fruit another seed. What intelligence inside of that seed is capable of producing another seed through a tree and a fruit? Find that intelligence within yourself and plug into it; that is how you become Awesome Again.

# 5. A FINAL WORD ON THE FOUNDATIONS OF AWESOMENESS

## a. Difficulties Are Normal

Over the years, I have seen men struggle with three ideas related to this program:

1. The attempt to understand everything in the Foundations of Awesomeness section prior to working on the actual Seven Steps.

   The solution to this struggle is to resist the temptation to get hung up on the details here, particularly if they seem confusing to you at first. Look over this section, grab what suits you, and move on to the Seven Steps. Some men may want more background materials and references than what is included here. If you are that man, know that in your personal portal at www.flaviolife.com/aa, you will find many additional resources and information.

2. The temptation to dismiss a Step needed to become Awesome Again by thinking, *Oh, I knew that.*

The solution to this temptation is to recognize the importance of actually accomplishing each of these Seven Steps, not just knowing about them. The explanations about the workings of the subconscious mind were included here precisely to help you accomplish what you already know but may not have done. These Seven Steps will only happen if you change your mind about yourself at the level of the subconscious. To that end, you will find included in your personal portal at www.flaviolife.com/aa, a number of guided meditations that will help you make the change you need at the level of the mind where change needs to happen for you to become Awesome Again.

3. The delay in results. Things may not happen as fast as you would like them to. If you are dealing with addiction and excess weight, you may have some difficult and frustrating days on your journey.

   The solution to this struggle is to know that you are not alone on this journey, for I am also on this journey with you. You are not alone. Learn to take one day at time and develop gratitude for all days, those you think were good and those you did not think were so good, because you can learn something from each.

In your personal portal at www.flaviolife.com/aa, there is space for you to post questions and concerns. You will find that we are one large brotherhood, all on our individual journey to become Awesome Again, but all supporting and appreciating one another.

We are all here to serve one another, to help one another succeed. You do not have to suffer alone anymore. You see, it is really important that you realize this: you are not alone on your journey. If you simply reach out, you will find help, support, and encouragement. You will also find an occasional brother on the path to Awesomeness who loves you enough to remind you that you can do better. Bless that brother and let us all become better together.

## b. Go Ahead and Be Awesome

You deserve my respect, admiration, and, above all, my deepest gratitude, for getting this far into your journey to become Awesome Again.

I specially want to thank you for the opportunity to share these ideas with you. You give my life meaning by reading these words and actually becoming Awesome Again. It is important for a man to have a sense of mission, a sense of purpose.

Once I had my own Awakening, I found a Purpose and a Mission, which is to help people change their minds about themselves so they can be who they really are. This is what I do. This is my purpose. This is my mission.

The best thing you can do for yourself and anyone you care about is to become Awesome Again, to find your purpose, your mission, your passion. For now, your mission is to study the Seven Steps in the next section of the book and make sure that you actually accomplish them all.

I want you to become Awesome Again, so that you too can experience the joy that you so much deserve.

## c. Time for What You Will Actually Do

Next, you will read about the Seven Steps you must take to become Awesome Again. This list of Seven Steps is very carefully crafted. The list can be much longer than Seven Steps, and include steps that are laborious yet not necessary to become Awesome Again. On the other hand, the list could be shorter and miss steps that are necessary for you to become Awesome Again. The magic of the next section is in selecting what are the most crucial steps you must take in order to become Awesome Again, and no more.

As you read about each step, you will naturally find them to be obvious, but please resist the temptation to dismiss the step, thinking that you got it. Each of these steps is easy to understand but, in some cases, difficult to achieve because the change required is at the level of the subconscious mind.

To that end, you will find in your personal portal at www.flaviolife.com/aa, a number of guided meditations specifically prepared for you to accomplish each step in the series. The guided meditations will have an effect at the level of the subconscious mind, not the intellect. You may already know all there is to know about each step, but the guided meditations are not meant to inform you, they are meant to help you achieve a change in feelings, thoughts, and behaviors that will last a lifetime and keep on producing improvements.

Yes, you will notice that, although we will focus on Seven specific Steps on your journey to become Awesome Again, many other benefits will be realized as you discover derivatives of each step. As an example, we do not discuss *increasing mental concentration* as one of the steps, but you will find that as you come to sleep better, your ability to focus and concentrate will improve dramatically, making you a more productive man.

Time to get to work and become Awesome Again. Good luck, men!

# PART 3

# SEVEN STEPS TO BECOME AWESOME AGAIN

# 1. INTRODUCTION

Each Step presented here is a mental shift that results from paying attention to an area or function of your life. Each Step is a shift in your "awareness."

When you become deeply aware of something, no behavioral prescriptions are needed; no one needs to tell you what to do. When a man becomes aware of a need in someone he loves, he naturally does what needs to be done to satisfy that need. Awareness of a need elicits the right choices and behaviors from a man naturally.

Although each actual Step is a change in your awareness, each will elicit many actions from you.

You will become Awesome Again by becoming aware of the importance of each of these areas or functions in your life; you will work on and develop each of these seven areas of your life each day. As your awareness of the importance of each of these Steps grows, you will notice two things happening:

1. You will continue to improve each of the seven functions, making you more Awesome each day.
2. Other areas of your life that are not mentioned here stand out naturally as needing your attention. You will

find that areas of your life we have not discussed here improve naturally as you embark on a journey to gradually master each of the Seven Steps. Think of how you see the walls in the house once you change the floor; it now needs painting. When you improve one thing, you see the need to improve everything else.

Men tend to be task and action oriented. Men love to have a mission, to have something to do, to accomplish. Men are designed to solve specific problems, one at a time, and then move on to the next need. A man's mind is good at focusing on one task or action at a time. Men tend to have a single focus, and the focus tends to be on actions more than on mind shifts. Yet actions come from the mind, so taking the sorts of actions that will make you Awesome Again requires a mental shift first.

This program is easy to follow. You will find everything you need to succeed here and in your personal portal at www.flaviolife.com/aa. I am confident that you will do absolutely great with these Seven Steps on your way to becoming Awesome Again because I know you are willing to do the work required.

The Seven Steps to become Awesome Again are:

1. Talk it out.
2. Quit all toxic substances.
3. Sleep well.
4. Mind your health.
5. Release negativity.

6. Upgrade yourself.
7. Contemplate your life.

You may wonder why these Seven Steps and why not others, why not fewer or more Steps to become Awesome Again. I developed this program working mostly with one man at a time at my office over more than 20 years. In the beginning, I simply listened to the needs of men who wanted to become Awesome Again and noted their areas of primary concern. Later, I started testing what Steps were necessary and sufficient to create lasting change. When we introduced too many steps, they may have been interesting but not necessary to becoming Awesome Again. Conversely, when we decreased the number of proposed steps, something would be missing. Over the years, it became clear that if a man achieves these Seven Steps, he will become Awesome Again.

Each of the Seven Steps is presented as you may be feeling now, and as you could feel once you make the proposed changes. It is important for a man to have an ideal to pursue; therefore, in each step an ideal is presented.

Do not worry if you think you cannot achieve any ideal or any of the Seven Steps. What is important is that you follow the system to change your mind about each of these Seven Areas of your life. The system is composed of:

1. A brief description of each Step.
2. A parting thought, an invitation to "think about it".
3. An action step you can take immediately.

4. A guided meditation in your personal portal at www.flaviolife.com/aa, specifically designed to help you achieve that Step.

## *Think About It*

Start your journey to become Awesome Again by realizing that you must transform yourself. Many people depend on you, look up to you, and expect you to become Awesome Again. You are an inspiration to many people. Now it is time for you to step up your game and become the hero you know you are. Become the hero your loved ones need you to be. So, let us get to work!

## *What You Can Do Now*

You may want to read through the Seven Steps once to get a big picture of what the program is all about. Alternatively, you may want to study each Step carefully and make significant headway before moving on to the next Step. There is no right or wrong way to do this, but your intuition will guide you in the right direction. The important thing is to get to work right now.

When you are ready to execute each Step, you will need to schedule a few minutes each day to plan and act on each of the Seven Steps presented.

Decide now when you will actually do what needs to be done. Book some time with yourself each day to master each of the Seven Steps.

Log on to your personal portal at www.flaviolife.com/aa, where you will find your guided meditations. The guided meditations are an integral part of the program. The meditations are designed to help you change your mind about yourself, and to stay motivated.

# STEP 1: TALK IT OUT

*Men do not complain, whine or cry.*
*Nobody said life would be easy.*
*–Anonymous*

By the time you were a young adult, you had an idea of how to live your life. You thought this idea was all your own; you thought you came up with your own plan on how to create an Awesome Life for yourself. But you were deceived, not once but twice.

The plan you thought was all your own was actually instilled into you since before you were born. Most of that plan represents the supposed fixes to the frustrations of your parents and teachers. They drilled ideas into your head each day until you thought those ideas were your own. They were not. The first way in which you were deceived was by believing that someone else's ideas were your own.

The second level of deception has to do with the ideas themselves; they simply do not work. Think about it: what does a father teach his son most emphatically? What he learned from his mistakes. But your father did not have an opportunity to live his life over and test out his own ideas. Your father, parents, teachers, and elders thought they found answers to problems they had years earlier and instilled those answers into you as though they were absolute truths.

You accepted their ideas as truisms. You did what you thought was right. You worked hard. And here we are, working to become Awesome Again because you feel that you lost your edge. Something did not work. You did not fail; the promises failed you.

You are meant to be free and filled with joy. Yes, you are meant to work hard, but the definition of work has to be adjusted. Your work is meant to be an expression of your passion, a hobby you get paid to do. Your work is meant to be your contribution to a better world. Your work must bring you a sense of dignity and even heroism.

Your body is meant to serve as a vehicle through which you work and experience joy. Your body is built to work and to love, to contribute to the well-being of others. Your body is meant to be healthy and strong.

As you read about being deceived and having lost your edge, and about how two aspects of your life are meant to be, it may occur to you that it is time to act on your own ideals. But what ideals are yours? What ideals were installed in your mind as though they are yours? You need to sort this out by talking it out with the right person.

If you have lost your edge, if you are not as Awesome as you could be or once were, you are not Talking Deeply. Perhaps you talk all day at work with clients and coworkers. Perhaps you have a significant other whom you see every day; but if you are not feeling Awesome, you are not Talking Deeply. You might be screaming all day, defending parts of yourself on one hand, or you might be very quiet, pretending that everything is okay while you are being eaten up on the inside, but you are not Deep Talking.

Deep Talking means opening up your heart with another human being, discovering who you truly are, and letting go of who you are not. In order for you to become Awesome Again, you are going to have to talk your heart and your emotions out. Two things happen when you Deep Talk:

1. You decompress, unload emotions and feelings, guilt and shame, frustrations and regrets that may have been weighing you down.

2. You sort your true identity out of the sea of ideas that you absorbed from others throughout your life. You discover who you truly are. You let go of who you are not.

Find a person skilled in Deep Talking. Find a friend, a therapist, or a counselor. Find a rabbi, priest, or minister. Find someone whom you can trust and actually talk out your feelings, emotions, and thoughts.

Deep Talking is not a one-shot deal; it is not an event, it is a process. It may take some time for you to see the value of Deep Talking because there may be a lot of accumulated frustrations within you. But you can learn to open up deeply. You will sort out who you are from what you have been told you are. You will incorporate into your life aspects of your nature that were neglected, and you will let go of features that do not belong to you.

This is deep stuff; it may take a while to achieve. Quick conversations without a follow up a few days afterwards do not lend themselves to the deepening required for these results to be achieved. Quick conversations barely scratch the surface of what is really going on within you.

Deep Talking takes learning, getting used to, and much trust in the process and the person you embarked on this mission with. It is imperative that you find someone trained in helping others explore who they are and open up deeply.

Because Deep Talking is an ongoing process, keep two things in mind:

1. It is okay to change interlocutors eventually, but make sure that you are going toward a more challenging interaction, instead of running away from a difficulty.

2. Schedule time and meet with your interlocutor preferably twice each week. The meeting can be online or phone. Read the remaining Steps needed to become Awesome Again and decide what topics you want to discuss during your sessions. Actively work on the other steps even while your Deep Talk sessions continue.

Talking it all out deeply is the first step in becoming Awesome Again. This step may be tricky for some men who are not used to Deep Talking, but it can be mastered with practice and the proper guidance. Learn to Deep Talk and become Awesome Again.

## *Think About It*

How often have you wished you could be totally open and honest with someone and get honest feedback with no judgment? You probably can remember many times wishing for that type of conversation. Your wish means that you recognize the value of Deep Talking. Learn to Deep Talk well because it will help you become Awesome Again.

## *What You Can Do Now*

Make a list of all the potential people you could Deep Talk with: a friend, a spouse, a parent, a sibling, a therapist, a coach, a rabbi, a priest, or minister.

Go through your list, narrow it down to a few choices, tell each person what you need, and listen to their feedback. Choose one person and enter into an agreement with that person to begin working, to Deep Talk and sort out who you are, to sort out your own ideas from those of others.

I suggest you choose a person you can trust, not necessarily one you feel comfortable with initially. Specifically, you need to trust this person to:

1. Not judge you.
2. Listen Deeply, actively and attentively.
3. Have the ability to guide you into deeper portions of yourself.
4. Be free of secondary agendas.

5. Keep their own ideas out of the Deep Talk.

Get to work. Open your heart up, bare your soul, and question your thoughts and assumptions. It is okay to switch confidants later on, but you need to get started now. The talks need to be deep and frequent enough to actually get past the casual superficialities of social interactions.

Your goal is self-awareness; you need to know what parts of your life belong to you and what parts amount to an imitation of, or obedience to, other people. You need to sort out who you truly are, and, most importantly, you need to let go of who you are not.

Visit your personal portal at www.flaviolife.com/aa and use the guided meditation to help you with this Step. All instructions you need to use the guided meditations are in your personal portal.

# STEP 2: QUIT ALL TOXIC SUBSTANCES

*When the mind is unobstructed,*
*the result is truth.*
*–Anthony de Mello*

## *Introduction*

In order for you to become Awesome Again, you are going to have to quit all toxic substances. For some of you, this is a huge step because prescription or recreational drugs may be a big part of your life. If you think that quitting all toxic substances is too much of a task for you right now, keep the following ideas in mind as you read the rest of this chapter:

1. You are not alone! By now, or soon, you have your Deep Talks with the person you chose and trust. Even if that person cannot help you with addictions directly, they will support you on your journey to eliminate all toxic substances from your life.

2. You have massive support in your personal portal at www.flaviolife.com/aa. You have already paid for those resources when you purchased this book; use all of the resources frequently. Of particular importance in your personal portal are the guided meditations that will help you heal many aspects of your being.

3. You do not have to do all of this at once. Different Steps will be more difficult for different men because of what has been going on in your life. Do not worry if you do not think you can tackle this one for now; just know that this is one required Step to feel Awesome Again, and that you will get to it eventually. Some men have to make significant advances with several Steps before they can engage one particularly difficult Step for them. Trust yourself and know that you will eliminate all toxic substances from your life when you are ready to do so.

This is a big, polarizing, issue. Some men come to see me after doing extensive research on how much of a particular toxic substance is not too much for them; or how they actually need this or that poison to function.

The truth is that using toxic substances is costing you your own vitality. Sure, you get a benefit from the toxic substances you use, but their net contribution to the quality of your life is very negative. Their use is costing you your own sense of purpose, your life. No matter what kind of benefit you believe you receive, such as fun while drinking, when you add up all of the consequences, the net result is negative.

Denial is the ability to overlook the negative consequences of a behavior while pretending that the behavior only benefits you. When a man is in denial about the true cost of using a toxic substance, he only focuses on what he considers to be the benefit, while ignoring the negative consequences.

This Step on your journey to become Awesome Again will open your eyes to some of the consequences of using toxic substances that you may not have considered before. As you read these words, there will be a strange sense of urgency forming within you to quit all toxic substances.

There are four types of substances for you to consider eliminating from your life:

1. Physical substances: drugs of all types, alcohol, stimulants, such as coffee and energy drinks, sugar, and excess food. The topic of prescription medications is addressed separately.

2. Energetic substances: mostly electromagnetic radiation or pollution.

3. Mental substances: pornography, violence, gambling, and negativity (most news), and idle pastimes such as denigrating talk shows.

4. Spiritual substances: hatred, resentment, and ill feelings toward yourself or others.

Every type of substance assimilated affects all four of your main bodies, the physical, the energetic, the mental, and the spiritual. Furthermore, these bodies all interact with one another, sometimes magnifying the negative effect of a toxic substance.

## *Physical Substances*

Toxic physical substances, such as drugs, alcohol, stimulants, sugar, and excess food, rob you of your vitality in several ways. These substances have a primary effect, such as mood elevation, relaxation, stimulation, or a decrease in inhibition. While these primary effects may seem to be positive, since they are the supposed reason a person would consume them, they always occur at the expense of a secondary effect, the unwanted problem it causes. The secondary effect of a toxic substance can range from a headache all the way to death. The ternary effect is the energy the body must spend to rid itself of the toxicity. Enzymes must be synthesized, consuming precious nutrients and diverting blood supply from other areas of the body. The quaternary effect has to do with the often-unpredictable effects of mixing substances in the body. People are surprised when a friend who uses both stimulants and depressants simultaneously suddenly drops dead, for instance.

If you use any sort of drug or alcohol, you are well aware of how it is robbing you of vitality and precious resources. If you are not aware of the deleterious effects of drugs and alcohol by now, there is not much more I can say here, except that you need to eliminate them from your life if you are serious about being Awesome Again. There is no judgement here, simply the statement of something you already know. Some men struggle with drugs and alcohol, never quite eliminating them from their lives. If you are one of them, make sure that you seek specialized help for the addiction, and you will be fine.

Most stimulants, such as caffeine, are acids. People consume coffee to wake up, but the consequent acidity created predisposes the body to tooth and bone erosion, and a host of other maladies. Furthermore, excess coffee consumption hides the obvious fact that you are not resting enough. By hiding the deeper issue a toxic substance medicates, it is less likely that you will address the real problem.

Excess food and sugar are the main culprit behind one type of diabetes responsible for all kinds of problems, including death. A person who develops diabetes as a result of overeating becomes a slave to the illness. Even if an overeater averts diabetes, body weight and adiposity is likely to increase. Excess body weight and fat lowers testosterone and makes sex more difficult and less likely to happen. It is imperative that you adjust your weight on your way to becoming Awesome Again, and eliminating excess sugar and food is a critical part of that goal.

## *Energetic Substances*

Toxic energetic substances include all other types of substances discussed, physical, mental and spiritual, as well as excess electromagnetic radiation.

Every type of substance creates an energetic response in the energy body, which, if sustained over time, will lead to physical manifestations. To illustrate this point, think of an herb, for instance.

Since ancient times, people have used plants as medicine. The part of the plant used for the medicinal effect is not the physical, but the spirit of the plant. True herbalists understand how to extract the spirit (the energy) of the plant and fix it in preparations that can be administered to the sick as medicine. The art and science of herbalism, and the fantastic results achieved, is an interesting testament to the knowledge that there is an energetic component to physical substances.

Although I help people eliminate drugs and alcohol from their lives, I never work with a person while under the influence. Occasionally, someone will tell me not to cancel a session because they are no longer drunk or high, since it has been a certain number of hours since their last use. All we can do during those sessions is introduce the notion of energetic toxicity and book the next session.

I usually remind them that distilled alcohol is called "spirits" because of the spiritual effect if has on the person. Alcohol separates the lower functions of the mind from the higher aspects of consciousness. This explains the changes in behavior, and loss of inhibition, observed in the person who ingests alcohol.

While the physical body may have metabolized and excreted a good amount of a chemical, the energetic, mental, and spiritual effects of the use may last for weeks or years.

In your personal portal at www.flaviolife.com/aa, there are resources for you to read and learn more about the energetic effects of physical substances, including references to the important work of Doctor Edward Bach (1886 – 1936).

Light is a form of electromagnetic radiation in the visible range. Excess exposure to light at night inhibits melatonin secretion by the pineal gland, making sleep onset less likely. This is the most obvious example of the deleterious effect of excess electromagnetic radiation, EMR, often also called EMF for electromagnetic frequencies.

The science on the biological consequences of exposure to EMFs is incontrovertible. Microwaves are EMFs as well. Microwaves can agitate water molecules and cook meat. That is an extreme example of the biological consequence of exposure to EMFs. What remains to be determined, and nobody really knows for sure, is what constitutes a safe amount of exposure, and what a given person is actually exposed to. When you consider that we are exposed to radio and TV signals, cellphones, Wi-Fi routers, power lines, cosmic radiation particularly when you fly above the weather, and all kinds of other electronic devices, it is not easy to measure the total EMF load on one organism.

Two things are known though:

1. EMF exposure at the levels observed today is a new phenomenon, spanning no more than three generations.
2. Other genetic and biological adaptations observed in the past due to environmental changes took longer than three generations.

EMFs interact with biological tissues and the energetic body. In excess, EMF exposure can damage tissue. The best thing you can do for now is limit your exposure to EMFs. Do not live too close to a high-voltage power line, do not stare into a working microwave oven, do not sleep with your cell phone next to your head, do not spend all day next to a Wi-Fi router.

### *Mental Substances*

Toxic mental substances include pornography, violence, gambling, negativity, and much of what happens during periods of mental idleness.

If you are in a relationship, the use of pornography will degrade it. A few men have told me that their women enjoyed and encouraged the use of pornography during periods of intimacy. Every man who has told me this ended up divorced. If you are not in a relationship, but want one, know that using pornography "meanwhile" is keeping you single.

The use of pornography degrades the man who consumes it, the people who produce it, and the man's partner if he has one. This degradation occurs because when a man becomes aroused by watching porn, in the mental world, it is as if he were having sex with those people: men and women.

The use of pornography is also directly linked with sexual arousal disorder or the inability to have sex with a human being without pornography.

Sex, in time, makes you a bit more like the person you have sex with. When you have lots of mental sex with many people, such as in the use of pornography, you become more like the people you watch. This accounts for the anxiety and isolation that some men report feeling once porn becomes a part of their lives. It would be better for you to build a satisfying relationship with one partner on your way to becoming Awesome Again.

Watching television or the internet with an idle mind to relax puts you in a receptive state to the emotional suggestions offered in the programming you consume. Thus, if you watch violence, negativity, or content that denigrates any other human being, you are accepting those behaviors as hypnotic suggestions of how to behave in similar situations.

These are examples of toxic mental substances because their consumption degrades you and is linked with behaviors that bring you, and those around you, problems. The link between content consumed and later behavior in children has been well documented. Among adults, you see copycat crimes after popular movies air, and behaviors similar to those portrayed in video games among avid players.

Eliminating these sorts of toxic mental substances from your life will definitely improve its quality. We once conducted a small, informal study at the office. I asked 10 people who called me about the symptoms of depression to quit watching or listening to the news for one week. At the end of that week, all people told me they felt a little better.

## *Spiritual Substances*

Any form of resentment, ill feelings toward yourself or others, amounts to mental, energetic, and physical poison. Think of the word "resentment" as "re" and "sentiment." When you resent, you feel the same thing over and over again. Psychologically, all resentment is rooted in self-resentment for having done or not done something that you now regret. As such, resentment is an unconscious attempt to undo the past while, in a way, blaming yourself for and regretting that past.

It is healthy to learn from past mistakes. Learning from the past requires careful consideration and pondering of past decisions and events. But when you learn from your past, you do not resent, which means that resentment amounts to a resistance to learning or acceptance.

When you resent, regardless of whom or why, your body prepares for battle in what Walter Bradford Cannon (1871 – 1945) called the fight or flight, or stress response. The stress response is nature's way of increasing the possibility of survival in a life-or-death situation, but if sustained over time, the stress response will degrade your health in short order.

The most effective way I have seen at the office to help a man relax, decrease stress, and sleep better is to eliminate or decrease resentment. Here, I describe resentment as spiritual toxicity because resentment is analogous to hatred, and hatred is analogous to death or killing in the spiritual realm. When we hate someone, even ourselves, it is as though we are killing them a little at a time.

The antidote to resentment is forgiveness. There is a lot more to forgiveness in a further Step. For now, begin to work on eliminating all toxic substances from your life.

## *Prescription Medications*

The attending physician at my internal medicine rotation in medical school used to drill into us the importance of a medication review with each patient, at each visit. This experienced physician estimated that, among elderly patients, up to 70% of all complaints could be traced to medication mismanagement.

The problem is that patients visit different physicians for different complaints and receive prescriptions from each. Often, medications have similar active ingredients increasing the effective dosage in the body, or plainly interact in a deleterious way. Furthermore, all medications produce some sort of secondary, unwanted side effects because similar cellular receptors in other parts of the body respond to the medication where it is not needed.

In general, it would be preferable not to use any medication, but medications also save lives. If you use any prescription medication, you must be prudent and exercise caution; and you need absolute transparency and honesty with your doctor.

The first thing to do is to find a great internal medicine physician and ask for a thorough medication review. If you are taking several medications, ask your doctor if you can stop taking anything, and what the consequences would be. Often, your doctor can offer a pathway to quitting a medication. For instance, if a man takes medication to lower blood pressure, but adjusts his weight, often the doctor will find that the medication is no longer needed and un-prescribe it.

I cannot emphasize enough the need and importance of talking to your doctor about medications before making any changes. In the psychiatric area, people experience severe problems when self-medicating or discontinuing medications without guidance from their doctors. A man with bipolar disorder, for instance, may feel good enough and quit his medications. That man may become severely depressed or manic, creating another set of problems that are far worse than the mild toxicity the medication imparted.

Please do yourself a favor if you use any prescription medication: talk to your doctor about each medication and ask for a pathway to safely quit or decrease dosages. But please: never change any medication regimen by yourself; always consult the appropriate licensed physician and work as a team on your health goals.

## *Think About It*

All toxic substances produce changes in mood or disposition, hide deeper problems that go unresolved, and create negative side effects. Quitting all toxic substances on your way to becoming Awesome Again will make a huge positive difference in your life.

In some cases, quitting becomes a challenge, but remember that you are not alone. You are going to find a renewed sense of hope and vitality by quitting toxic substances. Just by reading this far, you are making progress, and I am proud of you. You are well on your way to becoming Awesome Again.

## *What You Can Do Now*

Make a list of all the toxic substances you have been consuming.

Pay close attention to what and how you feel when you use each of these substances. Do you relax when you drink alcohol? Do you feel happy when you eat a sugary desert? Do you wake up when you drink coffee? Next to each toxic substance you consume write the effect it creates on you.

Now ask yourself a question: is there another way to achieve what I really want without using the toxic substance? For instance, if you use coffee to have more energy, ask yourself, how could I have more energy without drinking the coffee? Do this for each substance.

This is a great conversation to have with the confidant you selected in Step 1. As you learn to get a benefit without the toxic substance, you will no longer desire or consume that substance.

One by one, you will eliminate toxicity from your body, mind, and soul.

You will find a template you can use for this exercise, along with other suggestions and a guided meditation, in your personal portal at www.flaviolife.com/aa.

If you find it difficult to let go of a particular substance, trust that you are a man of your word and set a date to quit with the support of your confidant.

Talk to your health care provider about any medication you take; ask for a review of medications and the possibility of decreasing or eliminating some of them. Never alter a medication regimen without consulting your doctor.

# STEP 3: SLEEP WELL

*Each hour of sleep before midnight*
*equals two hours after midnight.*
*–Coach Johnson*

In order for you to become Awesome Again, you will need to sleep more or better.

When a man begins to feel that things are not going his way, he tends to want to figure things out on his own. The first consequence of a major preoccupation is loss of sleep, whether it is because he stays up later than usual, wakes up in the middle of the night, wakes up earlier than usual, or simply does not sleep deeply enough. When in trouble, men sleep less.

Now it is time to begin taking measures to improve the quality and quantity of your sleep. The National Sleep Foundation says that the average American is sleeping 1.5 hours less each night than in the late 1960s. Scientists link loss of sleep to the onset of many maladies, including premature aging.

Some men tell me that they do not need much sleep, that they are fine with three to four hours of sleep, as though that were evidence of their masculinity. A man who thinks that he only needs three to four hours of sleep is either overcaffeinated, overstimulated chemically, or functioning well below his true potential.

Becoming Awesome Again requires sleeping more and better; sleep quality requires the right combination of quantity and depth. During depression, for instance, a person may sleep for 12 hours yet feel tired all day; that happens because the person is not sleeping deeply enough.

Good sleep quality requires the right physical, mental, and spiritual environment. The creation of an environment conducive to good sleep is called sleep hygiene.

The physical environment in which you sleep should be quiet, dark, and cool. If your bedroom is not quiet, darkened, and cool, find a way to make it so. You will find in your personal portal at www.flaviolife.com/aa several ideas to help you achieve a good sleep environment, depending on the problem you are experiencing.

You need a good mattress that is right for you. You need a mattress that supports your body the right way. There are many types of mattresses on the market. You need to find one that is right for you. The size of the mattress matters, a mattress that is too small, particularly if you sleep with someone, may not be comfortable. The firmness of the mattress will determine how your body is supported, depending on your sleep position. Finally, the materials used in the mattress will determine its capacity to dissipate body heat; certain types of foam mattresses may feel good at the store for a few minutes in terms of support, but may feel too hot for you during the night.

Most large mattress stores have excellent sales associates who are trained to help you find the right mattress for you. If your bed is not comfortable, go into the best store you can find and talk to the most experienced sales professional there. A great mattress is a great investment in the quality of your sleep and, therefore, your life.

Remove as much electromagnetic radiation as you can from the vicinity of your bed, particularly your head area. Keep your phone charging away from your bed. Remove Wi-Fi routers from the bedroom or turn them off at night. Do not use alarm clocks that plug into the wall because they have transformers that emit EMFs. If you really need an alarm clock, do not use your cellular phone; get a battery-operated or wind-up one.

Experiment with different head orientations; turn your bed around such that your head points to the north, south, east, or west. Try each position for at least one week. You may be surprised to discover that sleep orientation actually makes a difference in the quality of your sleep.

Sleep position is a topic that gets much attention in the pediatric community. Should a baby sleep prone or supine, belly up or belly down? Actually, sleep position matters to adults as well. The ideal sleep position is supine, facing up, with no pillow. Try it out one day. This position does not feel comfortable for some men because they are not used to it; it feels unnatural, and because some men are overweight, they prefer a lateral or side sleep position. No matter your situation, work toward the ideal sleep position a little at a time, and watch your vitality returning.

The scientific explanation for why it is better to avoid excess food and alcohol for a while prior to going to sleep is a bit lengthy. Besides the physical discomfort associated with a full belly while lying down, the body redistributes blood during digestion, and there may be wide variations in blood glucose levels, which will affect sleep quality and may wake you up.

Unless you have specific medical conditions that require otherwise and are working with your physician on this matter, it is better to avoid all food for about 2 hours prior to going to sleep.

Some men enjoy the relaxation that alcohol creates, so they use it to go to sleep. It turns out that alcohol in your system makes it easier to fall asleep, but more difficult to stay asleep. If you ingest alcohol at night, you will feel sleepy, but you will wake up in the middle of the night. Overall, the sleep effect of alcohol is negative.

Some men need to urinate during the night, often because of an enlarged prostate. If you wake up at night to urinate, you need to talk to your physician first. If you have a prostate problem, please treat it. Additionally, consult the work of Dr. Dean Ornish, who has conducted extensive research on the effect of lifestyle modification on health.

All electronic devices with a screen emit light, or else you could not see them. Some readers do not emit light, but then you need ambient light to read them. Light emanating from electronic devices, such as TV, computers, laptops, cellphones, and tablets, inhibits the release of melatonin from the pineal gland. Melatonin is a hormone involved in sleep onset. If your eyes are experiencing too much light, particularly in the blue range, for one hour prior to going to sleep, melatonin levels will be low. Sleep onset will be delayed and you will be up later than usual until you "crash."

It is better for you to turn off all bright lights and all electronic screens one hour prior to going to sleep. This will naturally induce a peaceful sleep.

The mental environment in which you go to sleep also affects its quality. Fear of any type, even if unconscious, creates the sort of stress response in the body that keeps you from sleep. Any sort of threat, such as marital fights, the news on TV showing houses being robbed or the economy tanking, or even reading work emails in bed, will keep you up at night. These sorts of subjects create tension and fear, even if you are not aware of it. These subjects get your mind going, making you think, and that is not good for your sleep.

The last couple of hours in your day are winding down hours. Keep your mind relaxed and calm, which brings us to the spiritual environment in which you sleep. The word "spiritual" invokes the notion of personal beliefs, which vary from person to person. Not every man believes in prayer prior to sleep, but some do. Not every man meditates, but some do. Not every man journals, but some do. But one thing that benefits all people and has been scientifically shown to induce the quality of relaxation conducive to good sleep is *gratitude*.

Regardless of how you do it, who you thank, or what you feel grateful for, if you stimulate thoughts of gratitude within yourself prior to going to sleep, you will sleep better.

## *The Test for Good Sleep*

Here is how you know if you are sleeping well enough or enough hours. Ideally, you want to wake up at the same time seven days a week without any stimulation, without an alarm clock, feeling great. You want it to be easy for you to get out of bed; if it is, then you are sleeping enough and well.

If you have to drag your body out of bed during the week, load up on coffee to function, and if on the weekend or when you don't have to get up early or go to work, you sleep several hours longer than you do during work days, your body is exhausted and your sleep quality is poor. This condition is short-lived, it catches up with a man. The good news is that in order to become Awesome Again, you are going to sleep really well every night all night long.

Take care of whatever problems are preventing you from sleeping well, so that you can wake up every morning feeling Awesome, jump out of bed feeling great, without an alarm clock and at the same time every single day, meaning weekends and weekdays. This tells you that your body is not compensating on the weekends for lack of sleep during the week. That is how you know, that is the measure of whether or not you are sleeping enough and well.

Some men emphatically tell me that they learned to visualize a wake-up time, dispensing with the need for an alarm clock. It is quite possible to train yourself to wake up at a certain time with no external stimulation, but that is not the goal here. When you visualize a wake-up time, you are essentially using your mind as an "internal" alarm clock. But when do you wake up when you have nothing at all to do in the morning? You wake up when you have slept enough.

Here, we are talking about using your natural awakening to know that you are sleeping well enough. You know you are sleeping well enough when you wake up seven days a week at about the same time without an internal or external alarm. When that happens, you are sleeping well enough.

Since most men must wake up at a certain time to go to work, they should use the alarm clock as a backup. If the alarm clock is still waking you up, as opposed to you naturally waking up just before the alarm sounds, go to sleep 15 minutes earlier. Keep on adjusting your sleep time by no more than 15 minutes each week. Eventually, you will wake up each morning naturally. When that happens reliably you found how much sleep you really need.

Sleep requirements can, and often do, change. Diet, activity, and stress greatly affect sleep requirements. But the measurement for enough sleep remains the same: waking up seven mornings a week at about the same time without an alarm.

## *Think About It*

You know how good it feels to sleep well. You deserve to feel good. Do what it takes to give yourself the gift of a great night of sleep. Invest time and attention into the quality of your sleep, for it will pay you great dividends in terms of productivity during the day.

## *What You Can Do Now*

You need a sleep journal. The purpose of the sleep journal is to relate the quality of your day to the quality of your sleep. Having a great day requires a great night of sleep the night before, and improves sleep quality the next night. Day and night form a cycle, one affecting the other. In your journal, you will learn to note the factors, both during the day and night, that affect the quality of each.

You will find a guided meditation designed to help you sleep better in your personal portal at www.flaviolife.com/aa. All instructions you need to use the guided meditations are in your personal portal.

Work diligently on the quality of your sleep and you will become Awesome Again.

Here is a summary of suggestions for your quick reference:

1. Bedroom is quiet, dark, and cool.
2. You have the right mattress for you.
3. Minimize EMFs around your bed.
4. Find the best sleep orientation for you.
5. Work toward the ideal sleep position.
6. Avoid excess food prior to sleep.
7. Avoid alcohol prior to sleep.
8. Turn screens off and lower lights.
9. Avoid arguments and tension.
10. Practice gratitude.

# STEP 4: MIND YOUR HEALTH

---

*A sound mind in a sound body.*
*–Juvenal*

---

Each of these Seven Steps needed to become Awesome Again builds upon the previous, meaning that with every Step you take, the next one will seem easier for you. Much thought and experimentation was given to the sequence in which these Steps are presented. It turns out that going through this program, in the order presented here, works best for most men.

You found a person you can Deep Talk with. You have eliminated, or are working on eliminating, all toxic substances from your life. You are sleeping much better. How are you feeling by now? Depending on how much toxicity there was in your life, and depending on the topics you are tackling during your Deep Talks, you may be feeling miserable or great. Either way, I want you to focus on the task at hand; focus on being Awesome Again, focus on the outcome you want. We have more work to do.

Continue working on the previous three Steps as you embark on the fourth. This fourth Step may be huge for some men. If you visit a doctor once each year, you may feel tempted to skip over this Step, thinking that you are in good enough health. But please keep in mind that if you were feeling that you lost your edge and want to become Awesome Again, you cannot leave any stone unturned. Please pay attention to each Step, no matter where you think you are at on your journey.

The main focus of study in medical school, as it should be, is on pathology or disease. Every known disease has diagnostic criteria. Some diagnosed conditions can be treated; others must be managed because a cure is not known. Treatment and management can be paid for by insurance companies because a diagnosis has been established. In medical practice, therefore, diagnosis rules.

Some conditions, however, are known to lead to many diseases, yet are not considered diagnosable diseases themselves. If a condition that is detrimental to your health cannot be diagnosed as a disease, your doctor may counsel you to correct the condition, but not much time will be invested in it because the insurance company may not cover the cost of that conversation.

Smoking and excess alcohol consumption are examples of things every doctor in the United States asks patients about, suggests quitting, and moves on. Yet, these are two conditions that account for a host of other health problems. An even better example is excess body weight. In of itself, excess weight is not diagnosed as a disease until, unfortunately, the patient is in serious trouble. At that point, the person is diagnosed with morbid obesity; now, the insurance company may pay for treatment.

This discussion is important because there is a huge difference between not being diagnosed with a disease by your doctor and being in optimum health. Being Awesome Again requires being in the best health possible for you, not just being free of diagnosable diseases. A man may go to the doctor once a year and get a medical checkup. Unless he has specific complaints, the checkup will consist of listening to the heart and lungs, and a basic blood test. In the absence of a specific complaint by the patient, abnormal heart or lung sounds, or blood markers too far out of range, the person will receive a clean bill of health, even if his health is far from optimum.

You will begin Step 4 of your journey to become Awesome Again by talking to your physician, but that is just the beginning. You will need to work with other experts in order to optimize your health. Trust me, any investment you make in optimizing your health will return big dividends in terms of quality of life and enjoyment.

Your physician will give you a regular medical checkup and help you resolve any possible medical conditions discovered. Additionally, you will need a good dentist, possibly a periodontist, a personal trainer, and a nutritionist in order to achieve:

1. Optimum body weight and composition.
2. An exercise routine that builds and maintains muscle mass.
3. Effective nutrition.
4. Optimum oral health.
5. Elimination of inflammation.

A regular medical checkup includes blood exams, but it may not include a hormone panel and an inflammation panel; you need both, so ask your doctor for them even if you have to pay for them out of your pocket.

Hormones are chemicals that the body produces in minute quantities to control several functions over a long time. The doctor who studies hormones and treats hormonal problems is called an endocrinologist. Several hormones being out of range could contribute to the feeling that a man has lost his edge, including thyroid hormones and testosterone. Unless specifically directed by your endocrinologist, we do not suggest hormone replacement therapy (HRT) initially because as you adjust other health parameters, hormones may get into normal range. This is particularly true of testosterone. Furthermore, exogenous testosterone (T) tends to decrease natural T production by your body. In some cases, HRT is the best option for a man, but for many, it can wait since weight loss and increased muscle mass may bring it up naturally. Be sure to have a really frank conversation with your endocrinologist about the consequences of HRT before deciding on it.

Inflammation is a generic response of the body to injury or damage. The word “inflammation” literally means “in flames.” The five classic signs of inflammation are heat, pain, redness, swelling, and loss of function. You can have focal inflammation, such as in a sprained ankle, or systemic inflammation – meaning, inflammation all over the body. Systemic inflammation produces all kinds of symptoms that sometimes are treated as separate health conditions. The great news is that the body produces a number of chemicals, known as inflammation markers, that tell you and your doctor that inflammation is present in your body. The most common inflammation marker measured is CRP, or C-reactive protein, but it is not the only one known. In most cases, systemic inflammation can be eliminated, even without the exaggerated use of anti-inflammatories, by optimizing your health.

After the medical exam, you need a thorough dental exam. Depending on your situation, you may need extensive dental or periodontal work. Tooth decay is a huge health problem because cavities incubate dangerous pathogens that may even cause heart disease. Equally concerning is the area between teeth and gums. Sometimes that small space is colonized by bacteria that will in time erode the bone causing tooth loss. Finally, poor oral health causes halitosis, bad breath, which certainly impairs a man's ability to be Awesome. The good news is that your dentist is qualified to diagnose and treat some of these problems or to refer you to specialists in other cases. But any of these serious problems, if present in your mouth, can be resolved with the appropriate care, which you deserve.

Some private clients on this program are surprised by how much emphasis we place on the medical and dental consultations. There is a reason for this. It turns out that when men feel that they have lost their edge, they tend to neglect their health, particularly oral health. Often, the first sign of trouble is poor oral hygiene, such as not brushing their teeth as often or as well. You may have to revamp your oral hygiene routine; do whatever it takes on a daily basis to keep your body and mouth as healthy as possible.

Body weight and composition, exercise, and nutrition are different things, often requiring the assistance of different experts to optimize, but they are all intimately connected, in that one affects the other dramatically.

For years at the office, we have used the notion of your "ideal weight," something a person would come up with while in deep hypnotic trance. The idea being that your subconscious mind knows what is right for you. Once a person has an image in their minds of their bodies at the ideal weight, sometimes accompanied by a number of pounds or kilograms, we develop routines that lead to that result. Our job together is always to change the man's mind about himself so he can achieve his dreams. Achieving dreams, however, often requires ample use of other experts, such as physicians, personal trainers, physical therapists, and others.

This is how the term OHT, Optimum Health Team, originated among private clients at the office. We Deep Talk extensively about a man's true situation and assemble a team of experts who can assist in making his dreams a reality. We often review the OHT and sometimes add other experts as the need arises. The person you selected to Deep Talk with in Step 1 of this program can help you assemble the right OHT for your situation.

A common guideline used in medicine to gage the adequacy of body weight, and, indeed, part of the diagnosis of morbid obesity, is the Body Mass Index or BMI. The BMI is simply the ratio of a person's body weight in kilograms to the height in meters, squared. There are online calculators to find your BMI and more information in your personal portal at www.flaviolife.com/aa. Since your height does not change much as an adult, most variation in the BMI comes from body weight. There are technical limitations to the use of BMI as a determinant of ideal weight, but this tool is a good place to start finding what is right for your body.

Two men with the same height and weight will have the same BMI, but one can be lean and muscular, while the other may be fat, have frail bones, and little muscle mass. These hypothetical men are not equally healthy, but they would have the same BMI. This is why, in addition to BMI, you need to know what your body is made out of; the simplest test for that is the percent of your body weight made up of fat.

Basically, there are three ways of determining percent body fat: the immersion test, skin fold, and conductance or impedance tests. The immersion test involves determining the exact density of the body and calculating the relative proportion of lean-to-fat tissue. This method yields good results but it is laborious. The skin fold test involves folding the skin in several parts of the body, such as belly, under arms, and thighs, and measuring the thickness of the fold. This method is highly operator dependent, meaning that it is prone to errors. The conductance method runs a tiny electrical current through the body and measures something called the electrical impedance or conductance. These are electrical properties of tissues that differ between lean and fat tissue. This is the most convenient method available to determine body composition, but the results will depend on the quality of the device used.

Your personal trainer will most certainly have a device to measure your percent body fat and recommendations for where you should be for optimum health. The American Council on Exercise recommends body fat between 15% and 18% for optimum health, but do not be discouraged if you are far from that range. Becoming Awesome Again is a journey, not an event, but you will be happy with the results.

The amount of fat you carry in your body turns out to be much more important than simply what you look like. The ultimate precursor of testosterone is cholesterol. If the body is too low on fats, it will also be low on testosterone. On the other hand, visceral fat acts as a gland in that it expresses an enzyme called aromatase which converts testosterone into estrogens. Too much fat, therefore, also lowers testosterone.

It would seem logical to drop fat by simply eating less. When a man eats less, however, he may not get all of the nutrients he needs. There is a lot more to nutrition than calorie counting, hence the importance of working with a professional nutritionist who can also work with you on ideas on how to prepare novel meals that are tasty and nutritious.

You need to make sure that you are getting all of the micronutrients you need for optimum health. Often, the best way to be sure that you are taking in all of the nutrients needed is to take a high-quality supplement.

Exercise has two objectives: build and maintain muscle mass and decompression from the daily grind of life. As a man ages, even if he is active, he would experience age-related sarcopenia, or muscle loss. It is important to continue doing strength training at all ages in order to maintain muscle mass and overall health. Always keep in mind that exercise is not just for weight loss, although it works for that as well. You must exercise your body to improve muscle tone and mass, and to have fun.

Most people immediately associate exercise with the gym. Often, when I ask a man if he enjoys going to and spending time at the gym, he says "not really." It is important that you find an exercise routine that is fun for you, else you will not keep it up. Anything that causes you to strain your muscles and break a sweat qualifies as exercise; find what you enjoy and do it often.

## *Think About It*

Many men take better care of their things, such as cars, rifles, and caves, than they do of their bodies. There is no other way for you to be on this Earth other than through a functioning body. A body that no longer works and forces a man to lay on a hospital bed, limits his experience to that room only. When a man lands on the hospital bed and stays there for a long time, usually that is the result of years of neglect. Regardless of where you are at, you can begin to pay attention to these ideas and begin to improve your health. No matter where your health is now, if you are alive, you can improve it. Improving your health will improve your experience on this planet. Plus, you will have fun on your way to becoming Awesome Again.

## *What You Can Do Now*

Achieving your optimum health requires a team, your OHT. You already started building your OHT by reading this book and establishing a Deep Talk relationship with someone you trust. If you do not already have one, you will need a physician and a dentist on your OHT. Next, you will need a personal trainer and perhaps a nutritionist. Depending on where your health is, you may also need an occupational therapist and a physical therapist. A great massage therapist and an acupuncturist can also be invaluable on this journey.

It is important that you continue to assemble your team of collaborators. In your personal portal at www.flaviolife.com/aa, you will find a guided meditation that will encourage and motivate you to continue to work on your health.

# STEP 5: RELEASE NEGATIVITY

*Forgiveness is the only*
*workable path to happiness.*
*–A Course in Miracles*

To become Awesome Again, you are going to have to release negative feelings.

The sequence in which the Steps are presented is the result of much experience and testing. By the time you are ready to really work on Step 5, you have already established a relationship with someone you Deep Talk with, you have either quit or begun to quit all toxic substances, you are sleeping well or better than before, and you are taking measures to optimize your health. By now you know that, somewhere in there, you harbor negative feelings. You know this because during your work on the previous 4 Steps, you experienced negativity.

If there were no negativity within you, would you really have lost your edge or felt like you lost it?

Meet Phil who came to see me to lose weight. He was a successful architect, drove a luxury car, lived in a luxury home, was married, and had children. Phil was very pleasant to talk with and extremely knowledgeable on all subjects, including health. He was determined to build a large cathedral because he thought of it as his legacy as an architect. Phil was over 60 pounds overweight. Each night, well after dinner, he would raid the refrigerator and eat everything he could find, standing up almost within the open refrigerator.

No amount of talking would reveal any negativity or resentment. Phil was an awesome guy. I had heard of an investigation on corruption in the construction industry, where permits would be issued to large contractors but sometimes denied to smaller builders. I do not know what happened to those allegations but, since Phil was also a builder, I brought up the whole corruption conversation during one of our sessions. For the first time in weeks, Phil blushed and shifted his position on the chair as he talked about corruption in the construction world.

Our session together came to the usual, relaxing, guided meditation for peace until we met again 2 or 3 days later. To my surprise, this time, Phil went into a much deeper state of hypnosis than ever before. I offered Phil the simple hypnotic suggestion while in the state: You will become aware of the cause... we can talk about it...

We ended the session late as usual because it was so interesting to talk to Phil and exited together toward the office lobby. No one was there at the time. Phil looked at me and simply said, “My brother is an asshole and my mother still loves him.”

We talked for another hour standing in the lobby about his brother, his corrupt activities, and how their mother seemed to favor John, even though Phil was the good one. Until that moment, I did not even know that Phil had a brother; it never came up during our sessions.

Phil, the pleasant man who "for no reason" raided the refrigerator at night, held deep resentments toward his mother and his brother. Being a genuinely good man, Phil could not consciously reconcile his love and passionate nature with the resentment he held inside; so, as we all do, he buried those feelings deep into his subconscious mind. The only thing he could "see" was the excess weight, and the unexplainable raids to the refrigerator at night. Phil healed, adjusted his weight, and made peace with himself.

The point of this story is not about mothers, or brothers, or corruption. The point is that, often, we are not aware of the actual resentment; all we can see and feel are the consequences it creates.

As I discussed before, to resent is to feel again what we felt in the past. Because the mind is focused on the past when a man resents, his life cannot move on, leading to the feeling of being stuck or losing your edge.

A few men who harbor a lot of anger, hatred, and resentment are very vocal about their feelings. They hate life and will let you know how they feel. Most men, however, are great human beings, who, therefore, have a hard time reconciling their goodness with the ill feelings they harbor inside. When that happens, the resentment becomes relegated to the subconscious mind, and no amount of asking and talking will reveal the true source of their problem.

Resentment is a huge problem that needs to be eliminated before you can become Awesome Again. Resentment manifests in terms of anger, in terms of frustrations, in terms of loss of libido, and, eventually, the loss of your edge. The feeling that you are Awesome goes away; you feel dull. In order to become Awesome Again, you have to get rid of resentment.

There is only one antidote for resentment: forgiveness.

Forgiving one who really needs to be forgiven is not easy when you have resentment. If somebody did something to me, and I told you that I forgave the person, forgiving that person is relatively easy, but that is not what it takes to let go of resentment. In order to let go of resentment, you are going to have to forgive *yourself*. Ultimately, all resentment Is anchored in some sort of self-resentment. We resent ourselves for not having done or acted as we know we should have, for not doing what we should have done, or for having done what we know we should not have done in some way. Ultimately, all resentment is against our own selves.

Forgiveness is not a gift you give those who hurt and betray you; forgiveness is a gift you give yourself. Forgiving yourself and others is important because it frees you to now live your life with those who value and appreciate you.

Now, you can forgive yourself because you are well on your way to becoming Awesome Again.

## *Think About It*

What happened to you or what you did or did not do hurts a lot. It sometimes feels like a dagger right through your heart. I know how you feel, for I felt the same way, but what I found is that if I wanted to become Awesome Again, I would have to forgive others and myself. I am with you on this, and this is serious. You have to let go of resentment and regrets. We are together in this, you are not alone. You are not fighting this monster, this demon, alone; you have backup. You will forgive all the people in your life, including yourself, as a gift to you and to those who are counting on you to be their hero. Forgive yourself, please.

## *What You Can Do Now*

Take one moment to imagine how many men all over the world right now are on the same journey you are on to become Awesome Again. These men are all your buddies, and buddies understand one another. We help each other out. You are not alone, my friend; trust me. You have massive backup; trust me.

Go into your personal portal at www.flaviolife.com/aa now and do the guided meditation for forgiveness that we prepared for you.

# STEP 6: UPGRADE YOURSELF

*Living, Loving, and Learning.*
*–Leo Buscaglia*

To become Awesome Again, you will have to upgrade yourself.

As a kid in school, the teacher told you what to do and you did it to comply with what was expected of you. As a kid, you were rewarded with an upgrade; they moved you up one grade for doing as you were told.

Now, you are a man who wants to become Awesome Again. You will have to upgrade yourself. What does that mean? You are going to have to change grades; whatever grade of life you are living, you are going to have to study and work to move up a grade.

You will learn new skills, a new language, read more books, something that interests you, that is important to you.

Casual learning is not enough; you must become Awesome at something new that interests you. Focus on it and practice it, until you become Awesome at it.

If you were born in the 1950s, 60s or 70s, you are a baby boomer or Generation Xer and come from a world where the youth had to pay their dues. Basically, young people worked long and hard for very little pay, while an older elite collected most of the profits in any endeavor, simply because they were at the top of the heap, and because they had paid their dues when they were younger. Many men from these generations feel frustrated when they see men half their age making multiple times more money than they do and living a much better lifestyle than they do. Something in these men does not register as fair, as just.

The feeling of injustice brings massive action out of a man. Think about an old lady being robbed on the street; you see that and you immediately jump into action to assist the lady. Every man is a hero, and to act against an injustice is instinctive for men. However, men who are now working to become Awesome Again come from a generation that was conditioned to accept certain things as the way things were. These men grew up hearing stories about world wars, concentration camps, and massive bombings that, for the first time in history, obliterated entire countries.

What sort of action can one man take against a nuclear bomb? Against an evil empire? You see? These men, unbeknownst to them, unconsciously, were conditioned to lay low, to work hard, to put their noses to the grindstones of life, to not make waves, to take care of their families, to sacrifice themselves, to suffer quietly. These men were conditioned to trust and follow the system, lest the system swallows them into oblivion.

One consequence of this unconscious programming is that these men accepted a formula for success that had worked in previous generations: get an education, get a good job, work hard, and everything will be alright. Once "educated" these men would continue to learn on the job only what was required to be more productive for the corporations they served.

Suddenly, and it was quite sudden, these men found a new generation of young people who didn't care much about the way things had been. This new generation was solution-oriented. Where they saw an opportunity, a need, or a problem, they invented a solution that completely disrupted the old system with no apparent regard for the old system. As a consequence of their ingenuity, this generation became wildly successful in ways that some middle-aged men do not even understand.

When I began practicing hypnotherapy in the mid-1990s, older men came to see me feeling professionally insecure about their skill sets. They saw "kids" working with computers more effectively than they were able to, often felt intimidated by their younger counterparts, but did not quite know how to remedy the problem. Upgrading their skills back then often involved taking computer classes.

Today, the problem is quite different. The new Millennial generation is firmly implanted into our society. It is creating a very different world, and the reward structures of the past no longer apply. Upgrading yourself today means learning a whole new way of looking at life. Let me tell you two stories.

A man in his late 50s who was a public personality came to see me once. He had made a fortune up until the 1990s through television. His audience got older and kept watching television but dwindled both in numbers through death and attrition and in purchasing power. As his audience dwindled, he felt irrelevant, although still capable of making a contribution.

Another man, no older than 18, worked at a store where I went to buy a headset for my daughter. I asked him whether the headset I selected was a good headset. He told me that if I wanted a good headset, I should go to such and such store. I asked him whether the other store he promoted belonged to the same company he worked for. He said, "No, but they have good headsets there."

The first story illustrates stagnation and the tendency to expect rewards for accomplishments of long ago. That man worked extremely hard to upgrade himself until he could reach a new generation not just by paying for social media ads but also by actually connecting with them with a new message.

The second story illustrates a novel thought system. The thought of "promoting the competition" was uncommon when I was 18. But the new generation, which is different from the previous in many regards, functions based on collaboration and a whole different model of competition.

The Steps on your journey to become Awesome Again are designed to gradually help you upgrade yourself. Deep Talking to the right person is crucially important for your success. There can be no Awesomeness if the bodies, physical and mental, are intoxicated. Sleep is important not only for memory consolidation and deep learning but also for peak energy, enthusiasm, and optimum health, which you are already working on building. Clearly, letting go of resentments and negativity opens up the space for your upgrade as a human being. Understanding the new world and the new generation you are meant to guide and serve is a crucial step in becoming Awesome Again.

There is another sense in which you must upgrade yourself; you must upgrade your definition of manhood, your understanding of what it means to be a man.

One definition of "man" is genetic. If there is a "Y" chromosome in your DNA, you are a man. Another definition of "man" is physiological; if your genitalia are external, you are a man. Or, if you look like a man, you are a man. A subtler definition of man is "If you feel like a man, you are a man." With recent advances in cosmetic and gender reassignment surgery, you can see how these definitions do not necessarily align with one another. But this is not what I mean by upgrading your understanding of what it means to be a man. These can be very complex issues that affect some people, but not the issue we are dealing with now.

You know you are a man who wants to become Awesome Again. There is no question to you that your DNA has a "Y" chromosome, that your genitalia are external, that you look like a man, and that you feel like a man. The question is, do you function like a man? The question does not refer to sex; it refers to your function in society, family, and relationships. Before you can truly answer that question, you must upgrade your understanding of what a man's function is in this world.

In previous generations, a man's function was obvious: work. So long as a man worked and brought home the bacon, he was the man, no questions asked or needed. Most women now work, in some cases, making more money than their men. It probably should not be that way, but money issues lend themselves to power struggles and often destroy relationships. Gender roles have become meaningless as fathers care for babies, women work in construction, and they both do the dishes.

Unless you upgrade yourself and develop a solid understanding of what it means to be a man in today's world, you may end up not necessarily feeling like one. Can you see how that would gnaw at you deep in your guts and possibly lead to the feeling that you lost your edge?

Learn new skills to the point of being Awesome, learn the mindset of the new world, and upgrade your understanding of manhood in today's society. That is one important Step on your journey to become Awesome Again.

## *Think About It*

Look at the plants around you. They are all growing. Everything alive is growing. You felt at your best when you were growing the most. Upgrading yourself simply means moving toward growth again. As you begin to feel that you are growing, you begin to feel Awesome Again. People around you need you to be their hero, they need you to grow. Do not keep them waiting!

## *What You Can Do Now*

Start by making a bucket list, write all your wishes, everything you feel like doing or learning. Now divide a blank page into three columns: life skills, professional skills, and hobbies. Take your bucket list and place each item under the column you think it belongs. Pick one in each column and make plans to achieve that, starting today. In your personal portal at www.flaviolife.com/aa, you will find a powerful meditation prepared specially for you men who are ready to become Awesome Again. You may want to work with the guided meditations for several days, as this Step requires continuously upgrading yourself.

# STEP 7: CONTEMPLATE YOUR LIFE

*The unexamined life is not worth living.*
*–Socrates*

Congratulations, men! This is the final Step needed for you to become Awesome Again. I am proud of you for making it this far. This may be a quick read for you, or you may be studying these steps carefully. Wherever you are on your journey, I encourage you to visit your personal portal at www.flaviolife.com/aa and keep working on each of these Steps with the guided meditations until you actually feel Awesome Again. You deserve the results that this journey will bring into your life and the lives of those around you. Men, one more Step: let us get to work!

Throughout this book, you have read about your multiple bodies: the physical, energetic, mental and spiritual. Allow me to draw an analogy between physical existence and your inner life.

In order for you to exist physically, you have to buy food; call this "procurement." Once you have the food, you have to cook it; that is "preparation." Next, you eat the food; that is "ingestion." Food particles must be broken down inside your guts; that is called "digestion." Once everything is broken down, the body absorbs what it needs; that is "assimilation." Some of what you ate cannot be assimilated, plus the body must get rid of whatever it no longer needs; that is "elimination." When you eliminate waste and residues, the feeding cycle is complete. Food came from the earth, some of it stayed in your body for as long as it needed it, and some of it went back to the earth, completing the cycle:

1. Procurement.
2. Preparation.
3. Ingestion.
4. Digestion.
5. Assimilation.
6. Elimination.

Being Awesome Again requires that your mental and emotional life follows the same cycle. Let us use the mental and emotional experience of a vacation to illustrate this analogy.

When you acquire the resources to go on vacation, you are procuring the experience. When you plan the details of the vacation, you are preparing it. When you are on vacation, living the experience, you are ingesting it. When you break down your vacation into experiences, you are digesting it. When you incorporate the joy experienced and the lessons learned, you are assimilating the vacation. Finally, when you let go of the inevitable frustrations inherent in any human experience, you are eliminating.

Every experience follows that same cycle. Most men are great at steps 1, 2 and 3, or procurement, preparation and ingestion. Elimination is very important; it corresponds to Step 5 of the Awesome Again program: releasing negativity. Most men, however, need help with digestion and assimilation, which, in this context, we call "contemplation." In order to become Awesome Again you will need to contemplate your life.

Once you live an experience, such as each day of your life, it is important to "digest" the day. In organic digestion, food is disassembled into tiny particles the body can use or reject. Here you will need to "disassemble" your day and contemplate each experience lived. You will then consciously assimilate those emotions, lessons, and experiences that support your goals and direction in life and eliminate from your system any negativity you no longer need.

This conscious contemplation must be done nightly so that negativity does not accumulate.

Some of you may already do something like this but call it by a different name. Meditation, inner reflection, and prayer are some of the terms used, but the process essentially serves the same purpose.

Just as in the physical feeding cycle, we are being fed emotionally and mentally simply by living each day. When you contemplate your day and life prior to retiring each night you are completing the daily mental feeding cycle. Learn to contemplate your life, and you will feel Awesome Again soon.

Contemplating your day is not the same thing as ruminating, looping, or obsessing. This is how you contemplate your day effectively:

*Close your eyes and imagine you are watching a movie. This movie runs backwards, from the present to the past. Your mental movie starts when you close your eyes and ends when you opened your eyes this morning. You are "watching" your day in reverse. The mind is fast, so it only takes a few seconds or minutes to "see" your whole day. Watch this movie several times, always starting at the present and going to the moment when you woke up. Notice any tendency to skip, or get stuck in, sections of the movie. Gently ask yourself: what is it about this situation that I am not comfortable with? Resist the temptation to dwell on the actions of others; focus on your actions, feelings, and intentions. Tell yourself: there is a better way of handling this; when I wake up in the morning, I will have clarity and healing on this. Repeat this for each situation that you felt uncomfortable about and go to sleep. You don't need answers right now; you are simply instructing your subconscious mind to present you with answers in the form of dreams or awareness in the morning.*

And, as always, my deepest congratulations for wanting to be Awesome Again, and for working on yourself. You are my hero.

## *Think About It*

Would you feel comfortable if you did not eat or go to the bathroom for one whole day? You could live, but would you prefer that? Would you choose to let go of something so pleasant and good for you, such as eating and eliminating for days at a time? Sure, occasionally, a man may choose to fast for various reasons, but I am not talking about that kind of elective fasting. Most of us would not choose the pain that would result from an erratic eating and eliminating pattern. Why then would you not develop the same regularity with your mental and emotional life? Feed your mind and emotions each day and, at the end of the day, be sure to release what no longer works for you so that you can be Awesome Again and remain Awesome.

## *What You Can Do Now*

Pay attention to everything that happens during your day; observe with dispassionate interest everything that happens. Find a moment every single night, preferably before going to sleep, close your eyes, take a moment to be with yourself, and God if you choose, and, from that place of unity where you feel one with everyone and everything, go through your day again in your mind. Make peace with what happened. What did you learn? What did you get from living today? What do you have to release? What or whom do you have to forgive?

The best way to get into this habit is building it with a guided meditation that you can find in your personal portal at www.flaviolife.com/aa. This meditation was specially prepared to help you contemplate your life and become Awesome Again.

## *Now You Know*

We have covered a lot of ground together. You learned about the Foundations of Awesomeness, and you learned about the Seven Steps necessary to become Awesome Again. These Steps have been carefully developed and tested to produce the best results for men who felt that they lost their edge, but who wanted to become Awesome Again.

The sequence suggested for you to work was carefully tuned to produce the best results. It is crucial that you develop a working relationship with someone you can Deep Talk with. The work you do within that relationship will help you eliminate toxic substances from your life. Eliminating toxic substances and your Deep Talks will improve sleep, even if it does not seem so at first. It would hardly make sense to work on optimum health if a man is still poisoning his body. But once he begins to get rid of toxicity, optimum health becomes a priority. Sleep and health will improve, and toxicity will decrease or end, only to a certain extent if a man continues to harbor negativity and resentments. Once you release resentments, you make room for all kinds of upgrades. Not only will you sharpen your current skills and develop new ones, but you will come to understand life itself, and your own place in it, at a higher level. Finally, you will develop a nightly process that will maximize growth and minimize disturbances to your Awesomeness.

Your personal portal at www.flaviolife.com/aa will continue to be your friend. The guided meditations are an integral part of this program, for they will help you change your mind about yourself almost effortlessly.

The changes described in each Step will happen naturally and become second nature to you as you continue to work with the guided meditations.

Finally, I will offer you some suggestions on developing morning and nightly routines that many men find useful. That is next.

# PART 4

# KEEPING THE CHANGES GOING FORWARD

# 1. INTRODUCTION

Most people have achieved great results in their lives only to discover that things went back to the way they were before their effortful transformation. You see this often with weight loss: a person will adjust their weight through a major restrictive diet, then, typically, something stressful happens, and they gain all the weight back.

Most men work hard on becoming Awesome Again. Transforming a life requires from several months to years to achieve. There is effort, money, and a huge time commitment involved in any transformation. The last thing you want is for things to slip back. You want not only your results to hold, but actually keep on getting better over time.

The way to achieve continuous improvement after a major transformation is through the installation of effective routines.

# 2. THE VALUE OF ROUTINES

A routine is something that happens automatically. There is not much thought involved in carrying out a routine. The value of a routine is precisely the low mental involvement needed for the routine to happen. Because the rational mind does not have to be as engaged when carrying out a routine, it can be free to carry out other functions.

Most people are not very productive in the morning or in the evening. In the morning, many people say that it takes them a while to get going and engage in whatever tasks they must do for the day. In the evening, most people claim they need to wind down, but usually end up wasting several hours before trying to sleep.

If you develop both a morning and an evening routine that work for you, and that support your desire to continue becoming ever more Awesome, your life will continue to improve long after your active engagement with this program.

## *Morning Routines*

If, for years, you have been waking up, brushing your teeth, making coffee, and reading the paper before taking a shower and getting dressed for work, you have a morning routine. But you must ask yourself what your return on your investment is, your ROI. You invested a portion of your morning, your day, a portion of your life really, and may have sabotaged it with the negativity you read about in the paper.

For the purpose of this discussion, your morning is defined as the period between opening your eyes upon awakening and becoming productive. Regardless of what you do for a living, when you engage your main activity for the day, your "morning" is over; now your "day" begins.

This definition is totally arbitrary, of course. I just use it here to illustrate the value of a morning routine. Suppose you wake at 6AM, are a bus driver, and start driving your route at 9AM. Your morning lasts 3 hours, from 6AM to 9AM. Every 8 work days, you have invested a full 24 hours of your life in your morning routine. What are you building for yourself during that enormous amount of time? How much are you taking away from yourself by your morning routine? Let us meet two hypothetical men.

Man number one sits in front of the television watching the morning news before going to work, sips on coffee trying to wake up enough to drive, swearing at slow and rude drivers, to a job he dreads. Man number two jumps out of bed, meditates for half an hour, swims for half an hour, reads for half an hour, eats a nutritious breakfast for half an hour, does house chores for 30 minutes and commutes to work for another 30 minutes while listening to an audiobook. Both mornings were 3 hours long, but clearly these two men will build very different lives.

The purpose of the morning routine is for you to rapidly engage in some sort of productive activity soon after waking so that you can set up your day to be more productive, so that you can build a better life for yourself and those around you.

However you decide to build your morning routine, and whatever activities you decide to include in it, make sure that it supports an awesomely productive day. In general, a great morning routine should include these three elements, in some way that works for you:

1. Physical exercise.
2. Reading or studying.
3. Visualization or meditation.

You can customize the contents of your morning routine, you can experiment with the order in which you do things in the morning, you can vary the length of your morning by waking up earlier or later, but one things is for sure: intentionally designing a morning routine that works for you will definitely improve the quality of your life.

## *Evening Routines*

For the purposes of this discussion, we define “evening” as the period between when your productive activity ends and the time you close your eyes and enter sleep. As an example, if you stop working at 5PM and actually sleep at 11PM, your “evening” is 6 hours long.

Just think of each day as having four blocks of time. Be aware that according to how you use each block of time each day, each year, you will be building your life. For those of you with a poetic flair, think of each period of the day as related to a season of the year:

1. Morning: spring.
2. Day: summer.
3. Evening: fall or autumn.
4. Night, sleep: winter.

Your evening has three primary purposes:

1. Your personal, social, and family life.
2. Housekeeping issues.
3. Preparing for restful and regenerative sleep.

Your evening is a great time to practice a hobby, catch up with extended family members and friends, relax, and take care of your family and spouse if you have one. If you do not have a spouse at this time but want one, working on getting a spouse can be a part of your evening routine.

No matter who you are, there are always chores that only you can do, even if it is a matter of personal hygiene and grooming. You may also have to pay bills, do laundry, and prepare food for the next day. You may have to help children with their homework, and bathe them. But at some point, you will be done with these tasks of living and loving.

Most men are great at the first two purposes for their evening routine; but the third purpose is going to determine the quality of your night, your next day, and, therefore, your life.

The third part of your evening routine must prepare you for restful sleep. The Second Step of the Awesome Again program explains several key aspects of regenerative sleep. But part of sleeping well is making good use of the time while your body is resting during sleep. Many men are surprised to consider that there is a purpose for sleep other than physiological.

Later on, you will do an exercise to define or refine your life's purpose. Whatever your understanding of your life's purpose is right now, take that as a standard. Imagine that it is an ideal to live by. Your understanding of your life's purpose will, itself, evolve and change, but for now, take it as an expression of your ideal.

Each evening, before sleeping, compare the day you just lived with your ideal. You will notice that, unless you lived a perfect day, "errors" will need to be corrected. Now visualize the next day as automatically incorporating those corrections from the previous days. You simply see in your mind's eye the new day automatically and effortlessly being lived free of the errors of the previous day. Your unconscious mind will carry out the actual changes and updates during the night.

This exercise is analogous to what happens in any automatic control system, such as the temperature control in a typical house. You have a set point; that is the desired temperature. You have a sensor, a thermometer that senses ambient temperature. You have a comparator, which generates an error signal, which is defined as the difference between the measured temperature and the set point. The error signal is fed into an actuator: the heater if the ambient temperature is low, or the cooler if the ambient temperature is high.

Your life's purpose is the set point, and just as the set point at home, it can change over time. The sensor is your memory, awareness and contemplation of the day just lived. The day just lived would be the ambient temperature. The comparator is your consciousness; the error signal is just a determination to be better tomorrow. The key is in the actuator; all you have to do is to feed the "error signal" into your subconscious mind right before sleeping. In the morning, you will naturally arise a better man than you were the day before. Your subconscious mind worked all night to make corrections in your ways while your body slept and rested.

# 3. PRODUCTIVITY AND EFFICIENCY

People generally regarded as successful and happy tend to be very productive and usually are looking for ways to be even more productive. You can become more productive, as the word says, by producing more. But producing what?

If a man makes more money by working longer hours, for instance, he is being more productive, he is producing more money. Most people would say that what they mean by being more productive is to make more money by working the same or fewer number of hours.

We use the word "efficiency" to denote the ratio of output of something desired to the input of what it took to produce the output. If, to get money out, you put time in, the ratio of the amount of money produced to the time invested is a measure of the efficiency, not productivity.

This is important not because of your choice of words. This is important because it will determine your life satisfaction, your sense of contentment with your life, later on.

Producing more of anything makes you more productive. Producing more of anything with the same or less input makes you more efficient. But what should you do? What sorts of activities should you invest your time in while on this Earth?

What areas should you be more productive in? Less productive? Think about habits you want to eliminate; you want your productivity in those areas to be zero.

The focus on higher productivity and efficiency without an accompanying focus on what one should become productive in, and efficient at, can lead to frustration. This is where the idea of a *purpose* comes in.

In general, a better life is a more productive and efficient life *that fulfills a purpose*. The emphasis on being more productive without questioning your life's purpose can lead to great frustration as you discover that you wasted your life on something that was not that important after all.

Once you develop a sense of purpose and determine what you want to produce in your life, start by being more efficient at it. Pay deep attention and focus on everything that happens when you are doing what you are doing, and notice if there are wasted actions or thoughts.

You increase efficiency by deeply studying each process in your life and removing from it wasted thoughts, which lead to wasted actions and words.

Things like procrastination, hesitation, lack of initiative, or the inability to complete tasks result from thoughts and later actions and words that are not aligned with your purpose.

# 4. YOUR PURPOSE

No matter how old you are, your future life, starting right now, is like a blank canvas. You can draw on that canvas anything you want, you can design your life any way you want it to be. Nobody knows how much time they have left on this earth, but, for the most part, you are free to determine how to invest the time you have left.

When I say that you are free to determine your future, people often respond by telling me about all of the obligations they have such as bills to pay and people to care for. Clearly, a man should always take care of his obligations, but were you forced to contract those obligations, or did you freely seek them? You entered into each obligation you now have by virtue of some type of agreement or contract, which can always be changed or renegotiated. These changes may take some time, such as feeding your child for another 18 years, but, eventually, all obligations cease.

The best life you can live will be one that fulfills your purpose. The following exercise will help you discover or sharpen your understanding of your life's purpose. This exercise must be done over a period of nine days.

Each of the following four days, write extensive answers to each of these questions. You must only consider one question per day, and write all that you can about each question. Do not look back; do not plan or edit your writing. Just write. Write freely. You can add to your answers during the day, but do not edit or delete anything. And do not move on to the next question until the next day. Answer the questions in the order they are asked.

Notice that the questions do not specify a timeframe intentionally. You can start thinking of the next 15 minutes, and move on to the rest of your life, for instance, or you can think globally in terms of a lifetime purpose. Here are the four questions:

1. What do I want to do?
2. What must I do?
3. What did I come here to do?
4. What do I choose to do?

Although these questions seem very similar, they are not. Considering and writing extensive answers to each of these questions causes you to reach into different parts of your being.

Asking yourself what you want to do, appeals to your desires, a part of us that is unquenchable and always changing. Asking yourself what you must do appeals to your sense of duty and obligation. This question takes you away from the throne of your kingdom and locks you into a position of compliance. Asking what you came to this Earth to do appeals to a grandiose sense of mission and, in some cases, self-importance, but still locks you into a position of compliance. The only question that leads you to freedom is "What do I choose to do?"

This exercise requires that you actually take on each question, on a separate day, and write extensive answers to each. Focus on each question and write answers to each. Writing answers is important to decrease looping, which happens when you only think and do not write about something. If you only thought deeply about the answers to these questions, your mind would find a few thoughts that felt comfortable because of familiarity and keep on repeating them within you.

On the fifth day, take your answer to question number 1 and remove any words or phrases that are not strictly related to the actual question. For instance, question number 1 asks about your desires, but if you find a phrase in your answer that refers to your obligations, remove it from that answer. Remove anything that is not strictly related to your desires. Do not add anything for now. Keep on cleaning up your answer throughout the day if you wish, but do not add to your answer and do not move on to the next answer until the following day.

Clean up the following three answers during the next three days. You will most likely end up with three short answers and one long answer. On the ninth day compare your four answers, contemplate all four of them together, side by side. Now write your life's purpose. Write it and look at your answer often.

Notice I did not explain how to go from "contemplating all four answers together" to "writing your life's purpose." I simply asked you to do it because you will be able to do it on the ninth day. Trust the power of your subconscious mind and the process to extract understanding from it. Simply begin to write your purpose and the words will flow out of your system.

Once you have your personal statement of purpose, check your routines to make sure that they support your purpose. Have fun with this process; make it light, but take it seriously.

# 5. GENEROSITY AND JUDGEMENT

If you had to pick one word to describe the perfect woman, what would that be? Beautiful? Sexy? Funny? There is one word that encompasses all of that and a lot more: graceful. A graceful woman is a blessing wherever she is. Grace applies to men as well, of course, but is there an equivalent word that would describe the perfect man?

I have talked deeply with thousands of women over more than 22 years of clinical practice. Without a doubt, all women I asked agree on this word to describe the perfect man. Granted, they do not all use this word, but they describe the concept. This does not mean that this word or characteristic is all a man needs to be "perfect," but it does mean that if you press a person to limit the description to one word, this word comes up most often: generosity. A good man is a generous man.

A generous man is always asking himself "What else can I give?" or "What else can I do?" or "How else can I serve?" A generous man is always looking to give instead of receiving in any situation.

It is normal and natural for a man to be generous, but not all men behave equally generously. What robs a man of his generosity is *judgement*. This can happen in at least two ways.

The first is when a man judges who deserves what and when; this man kills his generosity. Let go of the notion that you are even remotely capable of knowing who deserves what and give as much as possible to all around you. Give freely, and not just money to the homeless, although that too. Give smiles, say compliments, do favors, please your lady as much as she can take, provide abundantly for your children, and donate to charity and to your community.

The second is when a man invests. He does not give freely; he invests his energy and resources where he believes he can generate a return. If you are that man, you are suffering, but you can change. You can learn to give freely without looking for a return on your investment. The man who invests, in this sense, is not generous. He is ultimately not a good investor, and he is always miserably poor, no matter how much money he has in his accounts. The judgement behind the investor is that he does not have enough to give; therefore, he must dispense his resources carefully to avoid ending up empty. That judgement separates him from the unlimited abundance of the universe.

We do not know who deserves what from us; we may think we know, but we do not. We have preferences; we like certain people and do not like others as much, but that has nothing to do with who is deserving.

If you are known to be stingy, or a shrewd investor in your personal life, you also need to be more honest with yourself. Do you really believe everything you have comes from you? The universe is always providing abundantly, and you may be good at transforming opportunities into the resources you command. But there is always more where what you have comes from. Release the notion of a finite supply of resources, release the fear, for you deserve to be Awesome Again. True generosity does not seek a return on its investment.

Give more always. But do not only give materially; also give of your heart, from your essence. Be a giver always. If someone misuses what you gave them or if they scoff at your gifts, smile and give more. If a person spits on your face, wipe it off and keep on giving. Some people will be bothered by your light, so they will do their best to dim it; they simply cannot help it, for it is their nature. These people are your best teachers, for they help you discern what is real in you. Bless them and keep on giving.

Being generous, always giving and contributing, makes a man grow. Men sometimes ask me about giving money if they do not think they have a lot of it. I learned that when a man really wants to give from his heart, he always finds the resources to give. If you think you do not have enough, give more and you will have more to give.

# PART 5

# CONCLUSION

# 1. INTRODUCTION

Students and clients often believe that professors and therapists live perfect lives. Once you read my story, you will know that I have experienced pain and defeat. My story is not special; I share it with you, hoping that in feeling my own struggle and later victory, you know that I am just like you.

# 2. MY EXPERIENCE WITH THIS PROGRAM

For years, things in my life just happened. Jobs fell in my lap; a friend invited me to open the hypnotherapy office; and twice in my life, a woman called me on the phone, became my wife, and gave me children. I wanted to be an engineer since early childhood. When I graduated from college, someone called and offered me a job. I wanted to teach engineering at the university; a professor offered me a position teaching. I wanted to go to medical school; someone introduced me to the Dean, and I was admitted. I trusted the universe to provide what I needed and wanted, and I believe it did. I believed that our physical lives are reflections of our spiritual lives. I thought I was spiritual, so I accepted that the universe took care of me.

I had a great time as a doctorate candidate. I worked at several laboratories, went to and presented at several conferences, published a few papers, met some of the world's top scientists, met with the university president, received my doctorate, and still managed a few important pilgrimages.

By then my second daughter was about to be born. I was happily married, but my first wife was not. It took me 13 months to recover from the divorce that followed.

Parallel to my academic life, I was a student of mysticism, which brought me to hypnotherapy as a tool that could make meditations more effective.

The day came when my mentor on the mystical path died. For 20 years, my mentor and I had discussed his succession; I would continue the Work when he was physically gone. I had been reluctant to embrace that possibility because, to me, other candidates were better-qualified. There was no false humility there; I actually did not think that I was the right person for the Work, but my mentor insisted that being a true teacher was a matter of the heart, and that my heart, according to him, was in the right place.

At that point in my life, I did not think that my heart was in the right place at all. I was an unhappy divorced man with two wonderful children. I was a medical student and had just ended a second relationship after the first divorce. A massive global financial crisis made it difficult to keep the hypnotherapy office open, and I held a deep longing for one particular woman.

I always believed that there is one woman for one man for life, and that true marriages are preordained or prearranged by the Cosmic. The thought of meeting my true soulmate kept me going forward until I met a woman I thought was "The One."

This woman was different from all others I had ever met; it was as if she had already decided that she was "the one," that she was "ready for me," and that all I had to do was to "follow her program." Both she and the situation were really strange.

I lived a really strange marriage because, on one hand, I felt that I was in heaven with the "meant-to-be" soul-mate. On the other hand, her lies would never stop; from day one, in big things and small things, the lies never stopped. It was weird to live in a mind-bending reality where absolutely nothing was certain. Lies kept changing into other lies, but I always felt that, deep within, there was an underlying truth of deep love and belonging together "forever." I did not make up that feeling on my own; she constantly told me how much she loved me, and our nightly intimacy sessions were heavenly with promises exchanged and profound declarations of unconditional love.

I was annoying and judgmental toward her. I also discovered that we had an attachment style incompatibility. She was deep avoidant, I tended toward the anxious attachment style. By far, my biggest mistake as a husband was to "test" her love for me, something called "protest behavior" in attachment theory. This incompatibility can be worked out, of course, but she refused therapy and any type of meaningful communication, other than intimacy.

Eventually, the lies became more dangerous, involving the authorities, until it all blew up in a very odd betrayal and separation, theft and poisoning, 3 attempts to run me over with her car, and even the use of black magic to "neutralize" me.

Without a doubt, the demise of my second marriage was the biggest pain and failure of my life.

I walked out on and divorced the woman I thought was the love of my life, my forever soulmate. I was perfectly aware then that walking out would probably cost me my life because of the pain, but staying was killing me. Somehow, I had to choose between death and dying, and could not even discuss that with my own wife who was always busy, as she would say, "getting in her groove." I left, and my relationship with life itself completely broke down.

Do you see how absurd my own experience, my own life, is and has been?

I did not sleep at all for about three months once I left the conjugal home. I would doze off for a moment, then immediately jump up startled. There was massive anxiety nonstop with periods of frank panic. I lost 20 pounds within three weeks. Heart palpitations were so severe that I went for a cardiac workup; enzymes were not elevated, but there were extra, abnormal heartbeats.

Nine months after the initial breakdown of life and order as I knew it, I remembered having written this book some 18 months earlier. I found it on some forgotten hard drive, and looked at it to see if I could use anything in it to help myself.

The first version of this book was written after 21 years of helping other men become Awesome Again, but before I was broken and devastated myself.

The steps needed to become Awesome Again guided me, just as they had guided hundreds of other men at the office. I started Deep Talking with several therapists, coaches, and friends; worked on my sleep; decreased coffee and sugar intake; went to the doctor, dentist, and acupuncturist; and hired a personal trainer. I worked constantly on releasing pain and negativity; I started upgrading my skills and went back to contemplating my life and meditating. Meanwhile, I continued to teach the Foundations of Awesomeness and other powerful classes.

By late September 2019, several things were clear:

1. I was better than I had been before the breakdown; the Steps were working!

2. *Awesome Again* had to be published; I could not keep it to myself.

3. The original manuscript no longer reflected who I had become. I deleted the original manuscript and wrote a new one by the end of October 2019.

4. I still had a lot of work to do because I was "assaulted" by a "wave of doom and pain" at least once a day. These "waves" would last from 5 minutes to several hours, but by mid-October there were "wave-free" days, and I had learned to switch them off faster.

5. Most importantly, my heart had been opened.

I woke up most mornings between 2:30 and 5AM to write; my only alarm clock was my desire to share this message with you. As I wrote the manuscript, I noticed that the book took on a life of its own. It was no longer my book; it was a program from The All to all of us.

Without a doubt, the hardest part of the book to write was my story. The original manuscript did not have any references to my personal life, other than "I am a happy man," and "I found the love of my life." I decided to include parts of my story here for you to know that I am just like you; I was completely broken, and miraculously, by working diligently with the Seven Steps, came back to life.

The difficulty in writing the story was that I wanted to show you how crazy I was, how broken I was, my pain and suffering, how difficult it was for me to recover, how weak I really was, and what total devastation looked like, in case you have not experienced it yourself. But the major catalyst to my transformation included decisions made by another person, so it always seemed as if I were blaming her.

Even during the most difficult and darkest hour of my ordeal, during my darkest night, I never blamed anyone. I pray continuously for my second wife's well-being and happiness. I have never understood how a person can love someone one day and hate them the next. I loved my wife when we were married and love her the same way today. I pray for her the same way I prayed when we were married, and I feel the same way in my heart and soul.

Please keep in mind what I just told you as you read this story, for this is the best I could do to tell it without blame. Wherever you read blame into the story, please accept my apologies, for you are experiencing my own shortcomings as a man and as a writer.

I see other people differently now. Rather than seeing what was wrong with them, I see the person's struggle to come up with a better version of themselves day-by-day. I became patient. I became more agreeable with other people. I do not care to be right, quite the opposite. I now happily take the wrong spot if it pleases the other person. I say hello to people with joy, with a peace that I never knew before. The Seven Steps to become Awesome Again are working for me.

I now see every encounter as a holy encounter. The classes are more powerful, more impactful, more meaningful. I now look at others with admiration and respect.

I feel that I have a lot to share about becoming Awesome Again. Although I do not claim to know anything or have any special abilities, I know that I can help other men become Awesome

Again because I learned how to find the seed of Awesomeness within myself and, therefore, within every other person.

# 3. PLEASE CONSIDER MY INVITATION

It seems to me that we are living at a time when the Sacred Masculine is under attack just as the Sacred Feminine continues to be. Both men and women are missing out on the opportunity to live better lives because they are being bombarded with external ideals that take them away from themselves.

I help people change their minds about themselves so they can live Awesome lives. Helping a man be a better man is no different from helping a woman be a better woman, or anyone be a better version of themselves.

This is important because it seems to me that the only way to build a better world and solve the complex problems our society faces is to help one another become Awesome. In fact, I want to invite you to join me, for I have a vision:

1. I have a vision of a world where there is no killing, aggression, or violence. Crime will be seen as a form of mental illness to be cured, not as bad behavior to be punished.

2. Mental illness will receive the same attention and care as physical illness. Novel forms of mental therapy will

make it possible for all people to be free of emotional trauma, opening the way to live Awesome lives.

3. People will feel free to explore who they really are, be all that they want to be, while also respecting all other forms of life in the universe.

4. Work will be seen as an expression of who each individual is, not as labor that must be done in order to survive. All people will find deep meaning and satisfaction in their chosen work.

5. Major physical illnesses as we know them today will be extinct. The body will be seen as an extension of the soul; as such, physical illnesses will be prevented by catching them at the level of the unconscious before they have a chance to materialize.

6. The whole planet will look like a beautiful thriving garden. We will learn ever more sophisticated ways of living with and from the earth, while building a beautiful planet.

7. All people on the planet will have enough resources to live a life of dignity. This includes nutrition, health care, education, and a social environment conducive to growth and development.

I believe Awesome People will build this Awesome world. I believe you are an Awesome Man, so I invite you to join me.

Your first task, should you choose to join me, is to become Awesome Again. Be sure to let me know if you need anything along your journey, for you are not alone.

May God and the Ascended Masters Bless you and your life.

Flavio
October 2019

# 4. ABOUT THE AUTHOR

I met Flavio in 1991 soon after he left his engineering position to go to graduate school. We were colleagues on the mystical path, but he saw me as an assistant mentor, as my hair was already all white when he was in his mid 20's. I saw him graduate as a philosopher, and attended both his master and doctorate dissertation defense.

We travelled extensively together along with other friends on the path. We spent one day alone inside of the King's Chamber of the Great Pyramid in Egypt. We took turns meditating inside of the sarcophagus while the other kept guard as did the High Priests of yesteryear.

I always felt that I was called upon to look after Flavio, as our mutual mentor chose him to continue his mission when he left this world. Flavio was just a boy when his future was revealed to him. I saw Flavio struggle with the pull of his human nature and his spiritual inclination.

Flavio attended medical school during the worst financial crisis we had seen in a while. Despite the difficulties of running a professional practice and caring for his daughters, he stepped up when our mentor died and became a superb principal instructor of mystical philosophy.

I saw Flavio marry and divorce his first wife. I was around when each of his four children were born. I attended his second wedding. I was with Flavio soon after his second marriage ended. Flavio looked and felt like a ghost. He was in pain.

We talked about the demise of his second marriage. The pain was not about the loss of the wife, it was about the dark night of the soul it catalyzed. What was so certain suddenly vanished, leading Flavio to question everything he thought he knew.

Flavio had to face some of his past mistakes, and that created pain for him. The pain produced an intense catharsis that lasted over seven months, he later told me.

One day Flavio was simply a new man. He told me that The Master had told him that everything was in Devine Order, the ordeal was over, his transformation was complete. I knew that he had finally received the revelations he was waiting and working for all of his life. When I asked him about the revelations, he told me that he would share with everyone in an upcoming book called *Finding T.H.*

Flavio shares from his heart; his students marvel at the way he explains complex matters in simple language; I feel privileged to know Flavio and look forward to the book in which he recounts his own transformation.

Armandito

# 5. NOW A REQUEST FROM YOU

I am proud of you for wanting to become Awesome Again. You read the book and I am confident that you have been listening to the guided meditations in your personal portal at www.flaviolife.com/aa to install the Steps into your subconscious mind for permanent, positive change. The work you have done has earned you my respect and admiration, but more importantly, it makes you a better man.

Now, please leave me a helpful review on Amazon letting me know what you thought of the program. Your opinions will help make this program even more Awesome.

Thank you so much and be Awesome!

Flavio Ballerini

YOUR IDENTIFIER CODE: 01-2019-52777

Made in the USA
Columbia, SC
22 December 2019

85725271R00117